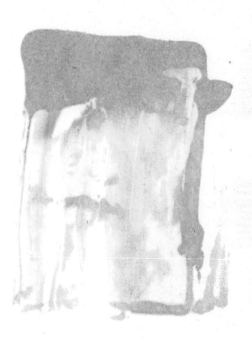

SKIN DEEP

Skin Deep

An introduction to
Skin Camouflage and Disfigurement Therapy

Doreen Savage Trust

with drawings by
Peter Trust

Foreword by
Oliver Gillie

Paul Harris Publishing, Edinburgh

First published 1977 by
PAUL HARRIS PUBLISHING
25 London Street, Edinburgh

© Doreen Savage Trust, 1977

ISBN 0 904505 20 0

Printed in Scotland by The Shetland Times Ltd.,
Lerwick, Shetland.

CONTENTS

DEDICATION

To my wonderful parents, Edith Torrie Duckett and Ernest Duckett, whose love and courage made it all possible; to my marvellous three children, Cassie, Caro and Michael for their devotion and understanding and to my lion-hearted Peter for his inspiration and support.

A personal note . . . from Peter Trust

A young girl over a quarter of a century ago had a dream. A dream that grew with the young girl into a reality. A dream greater than her knowledge. A dream so beautiful she was blinded by its brilliance to everything but the truth within that dream. The young girl became a woman, but the dream remained and with maturity she began, slowly and without fear, to make the dream into a reality.

Today, because of this young girl and her dream that all people should stand free and not be afraid to face the world, that people disfigured like herself should not shun or be shunned by a society often, in ignorance, afraid to question the reasons for their reactions; today, this woman, who most of you know as 'Doreen' or 'The Camouflage Lady' has made it possible, within her own limitations and limited means, for all people suffering disfigurement to find help: free help, safe help within the hospital and social structures throughout the U.K. Today, Doreen's dream is your reality.

To take this reality beyond the fragile limitations of a solitary person she needs help; your voice and thoughts and hands; in your own different ways help from each of you to make sure that her work is continued and developed — so that children shall never again need to question their right to receive help against the social pain of looking different.

FOREWORD

The rare albino animal born in the wilds must struggle to survive without camouflage. In the same way people need a type of camouflage, not to stalk a prey or escape a predator, but in order to look the same as their fellows and so pass freely among them and be accepted by them. The person who is physically different is as vulnerable to isolation and emotional deprivation as the wild animal without camouflage is to starvation.

A person's psychological development can be profoundly affected by the reactions of others to his or her physical appearance. The beautiful are sought after and surrounded with attentions while ugly, or just physically odd, people are shunned — at least until familiarity overcomes inhibitions. A small physical imperfection can be the source of a great deal of misery. Underneath the skin another person may be screaming for release.

I have a small birthmark which people now tell me often goes unnoticed. It seldom worries me now, yet I remember how often as a child I squirmed with embarrassment when other children pointed at my birthmark. 'What's wrong with your face?' was the question I had to answer so often — and I could never find the right words to say. There was a time when I did think of my face as being 'wrong' and it made me miserable and awkward with people.

I made a point of looking towards the left when I was photographed so that the large pinkish-purple blotch on my left cheek would not be recorded by the camera. And so I, at least, would not be troubled by seeing myself as others saw me.

Most adults play the same game and pretend that my birthmark does not exist, but occasionally I meet someone who cannot take their eyes off me. Sometimes they visibly recoil, with the result that any communication between us breaks down.

Almost always it's children who ask me about my face. I can now spot the question before it comes. If the child is with a parent there is often a whispered consultation and the parent can be seen attempting to forestall the question. By the time the question comes everybody is waiting in embarrassment for my answer. And I never know how to begin to explain it.

I went swimming recently with my two girls aged three and four. We were all in the duckling pool when a five-year-old girl, a stranger, came up and asked: 'What's that red mark on your face?' Undisturbed by adult embarrassment I was able to tell her: 'Well, it's like your eyes being blue — my skin is red. I was born like that.'

'My eyes are green,' she said.

When I was a teenager I used to think that I would grow a beard to hide my birth mark. But I never really liked beards, and somehow I decided that I did not like the idea of hiding. I thought that would, in effect, be an admission that something was 'wrong.' I was always aiming, I suppose, to try to accept myself as I was. I felt that to disguise it would just make me feel more vulnerable.

But you can never completely forget a deformity of the face — even a minor one. We constantly scrutinise the minutiae of other people's faces looking for clues to their feelings. And of course we try to communicate our feelings through our face. So any small imperfection of the face is magnified in importance.

Some birthmarks are too disturbing to others not to be disguised. People who are mutilated from birth with a bad hare-lip, a deformed nose or worse constantly suffer from the way their deformity interferes with normal relationships. Who can retain an entirely normal personality when everyone they meet will not look them in the eye for fear of embarrassment?

The face is the great focus of erotic interest, and people usually exchange signals of erotic recognition through the face long before they touch. And that is another reason, why a person with a deformed or ugly face may be as much a cripple as someone with only one leg. The difference is that someone with a crippled face does not get the sympathy of someone with a crippled leg.

Plastic surgery can change it, of course, but there are sometimes spiritual dangers in the search for physical perfection. People often project their feelings of inadequacy through their faces and expect a change of face to bring a change of mind. They confuse the face with the self.

Worse, a woman may so totally identify herself with her face that she cannot imagine living without the beauty she commanded as a young woman. And a man or woman may make the same mistake of loving the face and not the person. They may then say that their marriage depends on the perpetuation of their youthful good looks — and seek a surgical solution to their problem. This is a slippery slope which can end in mental breakdown in middle life if people cannot come to see their character and their face, or physique, as essentially different.

Personally, I would fear that I might lose a bit of myself if I were to get my face improved: I am not sure that I would be the same person inside. Without imperfections irritating my ego I might become disgustingly complacent. I cannot imagine it, but if people thought me so attractive that they competed to sit near me and talk to me then perhaps I would lose whatever curiosity I have about much of the world. The face is not the person but it leaves its reflection on the inner self.

In art and drama, beauty and virtue are easily confused. The hero and heroine are beautiful and the villains ugly. The villain can sometimes be recognised by some conventional sign. Until the beginning of this century it was seriously believed that criminals could be recognised by certain stigmata: low forehead, protruding ears, a face and physique more resembling an ape than a man.

Only rarely do I experience this kind of medieval reaction to my face. If I meet someone who approaches me from the right side, I may see his unguarded response when he sees my left side for the first time. Like a scientific experiment I can compare the difference.

Occasionally a flicker of shock — or even horror — passes across his face. Perhaps he wonders if these are the stigmata of a villain, or if something worse is concealed on my body beneath my clothes. Thank God I do not often see this sort of response. But I understand how, with people uglier or more marked than myself it can erode the mind like the drip of water on a stone.

Doreen Trust has devoted her life to trying to help people who are physically and mentally scarred. It is not only a matter of camouflage as she explains in her book. I recommend this book to everyone — not just to people who are physically different in some way. The problems of people with physical abnormalities illuminate the normally hidden connections between body and mind.

Oliver Gillie, Ph.D.,
Medical Correspondent,
The Sunday Times.

June 1977.

1: INTRODUCTION

'But Nurse, you haven't washed her face,' were my mother's first words as the midwife handed me to her. I now have three bonny children of my own and have experienced the waiting and natural anxieties that accompany the wonders of birth, and this has helped me, to understand my parent's feelings when I was born and, in turn, the feelings of the many other parents who have turned to me for help over the last two decades.

I often imagine the scene of my own birth. My parents, so young; both attractive, good looking people, deeply in love; excited, full of dreams and hopes for the future and the family they had planned.

I vividly recall the house we lived in and the room in which I was born. I can imagine my shy and gentle mother, rather bewildered; my father's three sisters keeping her company through the dark early morning hours, the arrival of the midwife, the talk, the baby clothes all set out warming by the old style coal fire, the little cot and everything absolutely right, prepared with such a joyful anticipation.

No-one present had ever seen a birthmark before, nor had they any idea what birthmarks were, apart that is, from half-remembered old-wives tales. One can imagine the young sisters clustered round my mother's bed, the encouraging family chit-chat, changing to a whispered consternation when I eventually arrived, and my mother's voice, asking why they were not showing her baby to her: my father's reaction, the dismay among relatives and friends. All the gladness gone, replaced with the worry, sadness and fear that inevitably take over, even when a baby is wanted and loved, as the realisation set in upon this happy family group, that I was badly disfigured.

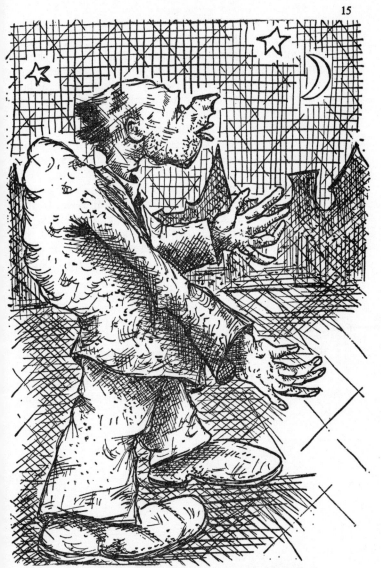

To look ugly is to be trapped in permanent public isolation.

It is easy, for those who have not encountered such a situation to be pious and preach that parents should be sensible, rational, and grateful in fact that their baby is not diseased or more grievously marked, but to talk like this, at the height of an emotional (and for the mother, physical also) crisis, to two young, newly marrieds, barely more than children themselves, unacquainted with suffering, sickness, physical deformity and full of hopes and dreams for their future family, is to be totally unrealistic.

I remained my parent's only child and their love, care and devotion are an endowment beyond any words that I can ever find. I was disfigured, but I was so lucky, for the constant sureness of my parents' love helped me through the many dark and depressing hurts I came to realise was the 'lot' of anyone growing up 'looking different'.

But what happened to the many others who were not so lucky? It was a question that overshadowed all my growing up, even as it deepened my own awareness and gratitude for the gladness I felt in just living and being.

I determined that someday, God willing, I would find the reasons why and do my utmost to alter things for other parents and their children. In my youthful idealism I had little idea of the battles and deprivations that lay ahead.

2: WHAT IS SKIN CAMOUFLAGE?

Disfigurement knows no frontiers

Any one of you reading this could be confronted with the problem of disfigurement, for accidents, diseases and crimes of violence are no respecters of age, person or status.

We live in an increasingly visual society, in which we have an excessive acceleration of the processes which create visual distinction. Additionally, the very nature of this society makes inevitable a rapid increase in the numbers of people, men, women and children who will become disfigured for, today, we must add to the usual incidence of congenital defects and acquired diseases, the ever increasing toll of road and industrial accidents, indiscriminate acts of terrorism and civil assault; large-scale injuries from horrific weapons of war, napalm and the like, as well as drug-induced abnormalities of many kinds.

Disfigurement is likely, therefore, to become one of the major problems of the twentieth century and yet, the Society of Skin Camouflage and Disfigurement Therapy, registered in Scotland, is the *only* organisation in the world whose *sole purpose* is to study the needs and problems of disfigured people and to offer support, encouragement, help and self-help as well as providing a platform for the exchange of ideas through its newsletter *Talkabout Camouflage*. Furthermore, this is the first and only book on disfigurement in total.

The ideas and knowledge from many disciplines and sources form and have formed the basis for the development of this new and specialised approach to the problems of disfigurement and it is hoped that this brief and

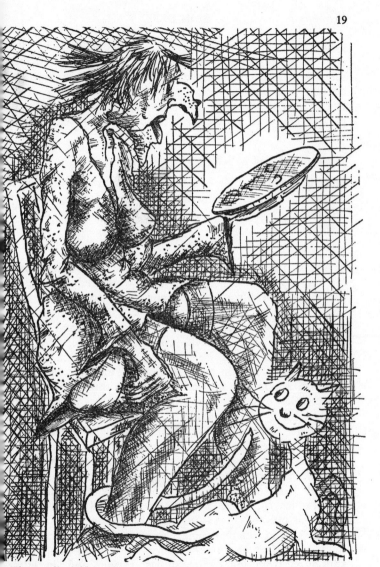

The small child in the street pulled her mother's arm and pointing at me said, 'Look Mummy, a real witch'.

generalised introduction to skin camouflage and the concept of disfigurement therapy will encourage further reading, thought and research, in addition to a personal concern and support for the work of The Society in its endeavours to establish a worldwide, specialised and supportive approach to the problems of looking and feeling different.

Background and beliefs

Disfigurement therapy can be defined as a *total* approach to the social and community problems of being visually different. It includes skin camouflage, the cosmetic component.

Background
The idea for a unified approach to such problems came out of my own experiences as a disfigured person, as the mother of three children and from my training and observations as a schoolteacher: it has been developed over some twenty years of study and research and the last fifteen years have seen the continuing development and clarification of these ideas through contact and consultation with persons in many disciplines, together with their practical application on well over twelve thousand patients.

Activities over the last fifteen years have included the establishment and conduct of Skin Camouflage Clinics, within the National Health Service, throughout the United Kingdom; intensive and incessant lobbying of the media in an attempt to stimulate awareness and discussion of this often taboo subject; talks and lectures both in the United Kingdom and overseas, and the assessment of, and replies to, some five to six thousand letters every year. All my activities — travels, correspondence, studies, research and campaigning, except for nominal and inadequate fees for some clinics, have been supported/ subsidised from my own earnings, savings and, in latter years, family deprivations.

In 1968/9 I went to the Department of Health and Social Security to plead for assistance to enable me to continue, and develop this work in the proper way, pointing out that, as a single individual, I was on the verge of becoming totally overwhelmed in every way in attempting to carry out, unaided, what was becoming in effect, a public service and that, without such help, my efficiency would be impaired in view of the ever increasing volume of demands for the service.

At the same time, I warned of the rapidly increasing danger of the commercial invasion and exploitation of the interest in the medical use of cosmetics created through my activities. I requested assistance in the establishment of a research and training programme, within the health and social services so that my own efforts over the years and the principles I had tried so hard to uphold in my work, could be continued and developed into a beneficial, ethically controlled structure to which end I had prepared and submitted for consideration various proposals as the possible basis for the further discussion of such a training programme.

It was suggested to me, in correspondence received from the Department of Health and Social Security in 1969 that I should form a Society as a platform for any such future developments and 1 duly formed the *Society of Skin Camouflage and Disfigurement Therapy*.

In the ensuing years, as predicted, commercial organisations were quick to realise that one aspect of my total approach to disfigurement, i.e. the *cosmetic component* could be taken out of context and had a vast profit potential, in the sale of covering products but, and more important, in the sale of related beauty products and treatments for *'Before* the cover cream' or *'After* the cover cream' or *'To use with* the covering creams' and, further, in the highly profitable beauty courses that could be organised to teach cosmetic cover techniques. The increasing interest in and demand for information and help, from the public and doctors, with the continued lack of support or assistance from official quarters, other than in encouraging words, permits, an unhappy state of affairs to flourish unabated, which irresponsibly seems to suggest that the solution to disfigurement problems can be found in a pot of cream and a little beauty care. A great deal of needless distress is created for those in need of proper care and further confusion created in the minds of those unable to perceive the difference between 'making-up' and making right.

However, such a situation in no way invalidates the progress of the last twenty years nor deflects the inevitable movement towards a greater understanding of disfigurement problems. I continue in my efforts to obtain the professional and administrative support that will enable a proper, ethical adequate Disfigurement Therapy Structure to be established, together with the creation of a climate of opinion which will enable future generations of disfigured people to find their full sense of identity.

> 'The problem of disfigurement is not that of the victim alone. It is the non-handicapped who by their negative and prejudiced attitudes help create and then perpetuate the handicap itself and the consequent burden of suffering. The surgical services must include both an awareness and application of the social, psychological, and cultural dimensions that have relevance for the understanding and total rehabilitation of the patient'.
> *John Marquis Converse, MD: Director of the Institute of Reconstructive Plastic Surgery, New York University Medical Center.*

Psychologist Doctor Thelma E. Brown survived a catastrophic car accident and became a facial mutilee. She wrote of her experience, from the time of the crash and emergency care to the completion of surgical repair and masterly plastic surgery reconstruction some three years later, and says in a chapter titled 'Ego in Distress' in Professor J. J. Longacre's book *Rehabilitation of the*

Facially Disfigured — Prevention of Irreversible Psychic Trauma by Early Reconstruction:

'What happens to this thing called 'Soul' that inner being or ego when your public and private image is displaced by a revolting caricature of things human? How do you face the future? How do you face yourself? Every such victim, if his brain is intact enough, must figuratively stand up and fight for the integrity of his protracted ego. Sooner or later he must, as I had to, grapple with alternatives and make a choice. And he had better choose wisely'.

Doctor Brown, with all the resources provided by an inter-disciplinary group added to her own knowledge and experience but, nevertheless, had a long, hard struggle to re-build her ego-strength. . . . for it is one thing to know and quite another effectively to apply what is known.

There are many forms of stress/disaster/handicap and many supportive principles apply to all, but, additionally, each type of problem requires its own special and specific procedures to be effective. I believe this to be true also for the problem of disfigurement.

Surgeons can perform miracles of healing and reconstruction but, in the fields of defect, disease and injury, there will be obvious limitations for many patients.

To date, attempts to re-establish such people have been based on the assumption that to disguise the defect and bring the person, albeit temporarily, back into the fold of what is the acceptable, though ambiguous, 'norm' will resolve the problem for both the disfigured and the non-disfigured. Such an approach recognises that to be distinctly different in form or function or both creates difficulties for observed and observer alike, but it increases the problem and confounds the solution for the greater benefit by far is to the non-disfigured who are so relieved of their responsibility in coming to terms with the various forms of disfigurement that are a part of any society. There is also an inherent danger in such an approach for as many things can be somewhat exaggerated for maximum media impact there is a tendency for the non-disfigured to be lulled into a false, unintentionally unfeeling complacency:

a   that plastic surgery (few people know the difference between cosmetic and essential surgery) is capable of achieving total perfection for all people, and

b   that a disfigured person so altered makes a complete and absolute adjustment to the change and *from that moment* is equal to any non-disfigured person.

A congenitally disfigured person will have been exposed to varying forms of reactions, as will have been his family, over many years and will have made a series of adjustments to survive which will have hardened over the years into fixed behaviour patterns. Suddenly removing the root cause of such behaviour patterns does not change overnight the person or behaviour patterns. It merely changes the person's visual appearance which in turn changes the reaction of the non-disfigured and so thrusts upon him an entirely new set of unexpected social adjustments and assessments.

It would be unreasonable to expect that a delinquent youth of, say 16, whose root cause of delinquency was poverty and domestic pressures, would on his own and without help or guidance become non - delinquent if suddenly placed in a palace. Indeed, the new circumstances imposed upon him could well intensify his problems and at best produce withdrawal from a now alien environment. There are many people who devote the whole of their lives to helping such delinquents to make these recognised and necessary adjustments. Yet, in the field of disfigurement alone, no such help is considered valid. Such reasoning would seem to be partly based on the nature of our culture that teaches us from the cradle not to stare and not to ask questions about people who look different and which creates a safety barrier between normal and abnormal people.

It follows from this that we rarely question the personal and social problems of such people and if we do so at all, dismiss them sympathetically; sympathy without understanding only serves to heighten the barriers.

It is ironic that help and research are endlessly forthcoming for alcoholism, drug-addiction, smoking, etc., despite the fact that these are self-applied abuses — whereas nobody asks to be maimed in a car crash, born disfigured, or become the victim of some indiscriminate mugging. 'It is a pity,' an eminent professor, himself disfigured, said to me recently, 'that we can't go out and throw bricks through a few windows to assume delinquency, for then the help we might need would soon be forthcoming.'

'Facial deformity which is rarely physically disabling presents ramifications far beyond those of the physically handicapped,' says a surgeon in *The Psycho-social Aspects of Facial Deformities*. It is nevertheless accepted that many requests for surgical procedures would be unlikely to produce long term benefit because of underlying neurotic tendencies and the Mayo Clinic recently warned surgeons: 'Considerable patience may be needed to make such people understand that the plastic surgeon cannot make a silk purse out of a sow's ear'.

Professor Frances Macgregor, in *Facial Deformities and Plastic Surgery* (the outcome of many years of research into the social implication of physical defect,) Paul Schilder and many others refer to the dangers of personality regression that can follow corrective operations on the face when facial blemishes have been used as the hook on which to hang all inadequacies and point the fact that as the face is often thought to *be* the self, in the mind's illogical way. The acquisition of a new, improved face is expected to bestow, automatically, a new, improved character and that unless self-improvement and restoration are accompanied by self-acceptance there will be little lasting benefit or contentment.

Similarly, it must be accepted that the cosmetic obliteration of defects can produce damaging emotional disturbance and, for some patients, is likely to *produce* problems, greater than those of the unconcealed defect.

John Liggett, in his book *The Human Face* draws attention to the fact that recent motivational research indicates that the search for social acceptance and the pursuit of the satisfactions of conformity are the strongest spur to the purchase of cosmetics but, more important, research also shows that there is an entirely unsuspected inhibition that militates against the use of cosmetics. Many women, it seems, do not want to regard themselves as the sort of people who would be prepared to adopt so much subterfuge, deceit and artificiality. Advertisers now seek to imply that no real deceit is involved; the purpose of cosmetics is not to apply a curtain of pretended beauty but rather to liberate the latent beauty within, by products which 'maximise', 'reveal' and 'make the most of your natural resources'. This is a doubly successful strategy which at once quells the conscience and flatters the ego.

When it is recognised that there are stresses for those who use cosmetics merely to enhance normality or to follow the latest fashion dictate, should we not ask what is the likely outcome not only for visually defective women, but also for the men and children who, increasingly in the age of the motor car and indiscriminate terrorist, become facial mutilees?

ROAD ACCIDENTS

Year	Total Accidents	Total Casualties	Serious	Slightly
1969	261,840	352,894	90,719	254,810
1970	267,457	363,368	93,499	262,370
1971	258,727	352,027	90,868	233,460
1972	265,186	359,792	91,342	260,671
1973	262,392	252,732	89,444	256,881

CRIMES OF VIOLENCE AGAINST THE PERSON

Year	Total
1969	37,810
1970	41,088
1971	47,036
1972	52,432
1973	61,299

INDUSTRIAL ACCIDENTS — MANUFACTURING INDUSTRIES

Year	Incidence per 100,000 employees
1970	670
1971	590

HOSPITAL IN-PATIENTS RESULTING FROM BURNS

Year	Total
1970	14,000

INDUSTRIAL DISEASES — CASES REPORTED

	1969	1970	1971	1972	1973
Lead poisoning	118	70	123	85	58
Other poisoning	55	44	29	25	21
Anthrax	4	3	—	—	1
Epitheliomatous ulceration	111	92	70	36	9
Chrome ulceration	121	89	89	130	117
Compressed air sickness	2	3	13	—	2
Gassing	281	341	304	295	280
Total	692	642	628	571	488

These figures are taken from the Central Statistical Office Review which can be found in Public Libraries

Does *not* include:

(1) Congenital defects, e.g. birthmarks, hare lip, etc.
(2) Acquired diseases, e.g. CDLE, Vitiligo, etc.
(3) Out-patient burn injuries and less grave injuries
(4) Drug-induced abnormalities, e.g. pregnancy chloasma, etc.

It is easy and therefore understandable to dismiss disfigurement problems, to reduce them to a pot of cream, but such a superficial approach indicates an inadequate understanding of underlying social factors. 'A little make-up here and there' is no solution to the problem of disfigurement any more than a trip to a toyshop to buy a toy would seriously be taken as a satisfactory solution for anyone in need of occupational therapy. A growing body of authoritative opinion agrees that such an approach can be irresponsible and liable to endanger the progress and well-being of the patient. *No* help is infinitely to be preferred to *any* help

Professor Goffman in his book *Stigma* subtitles this as 'Management of the Spoiled Identity'. There is a growing awareness of the need to understand how the security of the disfigured person is undermined and eroded when he is the object of morbid curiosity, furtive looks, manifestations of pity, ridicule and repulsion and Professor Longacre writes of the 'waste of energies which otherwise might have been channelled into more positive aspects of personality development' and of this disfigurement syndrome as 'detrimental to mental and emotional health'.

Doctor Margaret Mead, writing on disfigurement, regards our present largely unenlightened attitudes as being the result of, and perpetuated by, our western culture and feels (as does *The Society of Skin Camouflage*) the real progress will take place only when disfigurement, like many other once taboo but now acceptable subjects, is fully and unashamedly investigated and discussed.

A professor of rehabilitation recently said to me that it was no good giving a paraplegic a wheelchair — you must also show him how to use it and help him and others to understand and accept his situation. Similarly with disfigurement therapy.

> In Nature there is no blemish but the mind
> None can be called deformed but the unkind.
> *Shakespeare.*

Provision of help such as that which we try to provide does not exist except for our own activities. There is, *Psychiatric help,* but few disfigured people start out in need of this. There is, also, a frivolous, irresponsible 'hide it' approach, grossly commercialised very often, which can be responsible for many people needing psychiatric help at a later date and is a sad indication of the still widespread lack of comprehension of these problems. There is, however, no balanced and *total* approach to the problems of disfigurement except as is envisaged in the work of *The Society of Skin Camouflage and Disfigurement Therapy.*

Aims and purposes of The Society of Skin Camouflage and Disfigurement Therapy

1 To study the needs and problems of men, women and children who are disfigured.
2 To develop a greater understanding and awareness of these needs and problems in both the public and the medical and allied professions.
3 To establish a strong and vigorous national/international centre for training, treatment and research with administrative controls, committees and statutory bodies to support the Society in this work.
4 To provide a platform for the exchange of ideas and information through the newsletter *Talkabout Camouflage.*
5 To provide an international information service on the subject of Skin Camouflage and Disfigurement Therapy.
6 To develop further, the formation of social/discussion community groups throughout Scotland, the United Kingdom and internationally.
7 To develop further, patient correspondence groups.
8 To develop further, patient therapy groups in selected centres with particular reference to the formation of

camouflage play-groups for the under-five age group
and their parents.

9 To co-ordinate many separate techniques (e.g. prostheses) for the benefit of the patient and to develop
new techniques and preparations to simplify and improve the service for the patient.

10 To enforce an ethical code of practice to ensure professional safeguards and control of the professional
activities and conduct of members of the Society.

11 To affiliate the Society to an acceptable union or
association to safeguard the rights of members and to
have the Society, not individuals, recognised internationally.

12 To research, prepare and administer a continuous training programme and select suitable candidates for training from the following two categories:

a suitably qualified persons who would thereby gain
exemption from the preliminary stages of the training
course.

b persons with a satisfactory background who are
strongly motivated towards this work as a community
service, for example, ex-patients and the parents of
disfigured children.

13 To research and prepare notes, text books, case history
analyses and records for reference and training purposes.

14 To establish Skin Camouflage and Disfigurement Therapy
as a new Health Care Profession within our National
Health Service and freely and safely available to all
who are in need of care.

As you will see from the aims and purposes of *The Society
of Skin Camouflage,* research, understanding, information,
discussion contact and self-help form the basis of all that
we are trying to accomplish and we believe that this will
lead to a realignment of present cultural attitudes towards
physical deviation.

It was difficult for me to decide the order that these chapters should take, but, as almost everything I do and have done centres round the fact that I believe that 'people matter' so, inevitably perhaps, this is where I felt everything should begin — with 'people'. People with problems and people who have come through their problems. I hope that you will agree that I have my priorities right, for after all, the 'great humanity' that we talk about so grandly is just people — and their dreams and fears and hopes and love for each other. People like us.

So questions like 'Why Disfigurement Therapy?' and 'Why Skin Camouflage?' are answered better than by any words of mine, by the letters and Case Histories that follow, for the answers will be found in your own hearts as you read through them, and these are just a very few of the many hundreds of letters I receive daily from all over the world.

'I have hated my birthmark until my Mummy told me about you. I am looking forward to coming to see you'. Love from *Philip aged 7*.

'I am writing to you as I too have a port wine birthmark on my cheek and neck. I have only now plucked up the courage to write to you. I am 80 years old and all my life I have known the miseries this has caused me'.

'I last wrote to you in July 1974 concerning my three year old son who has a very large red birthmark on the left side of his face. I received a copy of your newsletter *Talkabout* and carried out your advice. Our own Doctor refused to arrange an appointment for my son to see a Specialist as I had already seen one in February and he had said there was nothing he could do. I then took my son to the local Children's Clinic. The Clinic Doctor just said that all he could do was arrange for my son to see a Psychiatrist if my son became mentally affected. So I am writing again in desperation to see if you can help me further because even at three years old, when people stop me and ask what's happened to my son's face or anyone discusses his birthmark and he can overhear, he tries to hide his face. He isn't just embarrassed, he appears to be ashamed of it. It appears that all he knows is that his face is different and people keep talking about it.'

'Enclosed please find a letter from my patient. She has been attending this clinic on and off for most of her life. I have known her since August last year. She is a very withdrawn girl and it is only in the last few months that she has been able to confide some of her problems to me. She does not easily trust people. I told her about your work and when I had finished gave her pen and paper to write to you. The look of hope made words unnecessary. I do hope that there will be something that can be done for her — my efforts at helping her to face the future will always be thwarted unless something is done'. *Educational Psychologist.*

'I have a patient who suffered burns of the chin and the front of the chest and upper thighs in 1963. She is now 13 years old and is a keen tap dancer and has been entering competitions but her scars are a serious handicap and she is very self-conscious about them. I should be most grateful if you could help this child'. *Professor of Paediatric Surgery.*

'My face is disfigured and I cannot go out on my own. People make signs behind my back and sneer. It is awful that they can be so cruel and ignorant. Every day seems to get worse. I cry myself to sleep every night. I am desperate'.

'Please help me. I have a daughter who was born with extodermal displasia. Amongst other things this means she has no sweat glands, thin hair, false teeth and no bridge to her nose. Two years ago at nearly thirteen she couldn't take the teasing at school any longer and started to withdraw from life spending long hours in her room and playing truant from school until it ended by her taking an overdose of tablets. We found her in time and *at last* people believed me— that we had a problem. Last year Greta had a plastic insert in her nose to build a bridge but it did not take and had to be removed. So then they said they would grow a roll of flesh from her arm on to her nose and this worked but, of course, it has left scars. At the hospital they told her to use cosmetics to cover the scars but unless she cakes it on this does not work and we have tried so many. Then I read about you. Greta is going to college now to try to make up for the year lost by being in and out of hospital but she still feels "different" and that people are looking at her. Young children come up to her and ask what she has done to her nose. At first she did not seem to mind so much but as time goes on she is withdrawing again and I am frightened. If she could hide the scars I know she would gain in confidence. Changing the face does not change the personality, I know, but in the desperate teenage years it can help. Please help me if you can'.

'We have a little boy attending this school whose face is almost completely covered by a birthmark. Although it doesn't worry him at the moment we feel that it will in a few years hence and we would like to help him in any way we can. I should be very grateful for any information that you can give us'. *Headmaster*.

'Until I read the article in today's *Daily Mirror* I didn't think anyone like yourself existed who could really feel compassion and understanding for those of us with the same handicap. Yes, that's what it is, a handicap. Who can imagine the sheer agony of mind one goes through over the years? In my case it is because I am scarred too, on both legs and both arms. I am unable to wear sleeveless dresses even in the hottest weather and I wear slacks nearly all the year round because I can't bear the stares and nudges from people wherever I go. I've taken my children to the beach only twice in their lives and even then I remained covered up and unable to join in their fun in the water. Over the years as my children have grown up I've become more and more like a recluse, preferring to stay in the shelter of my home. At first, it was for months at a time, now it's been three years since I went out socially with my husband. Naturally, my nerves have suffered, no one can stay cooped up like that without their health becoming affected'.

C

'I have just watched the programme on Grampian Television and the reference to your skills and I ask for your help. Please firstly excuse my writing as for the past few years my hand and legs have been affected by Multiple Sclerosis. This I have accepted and can live with although it is a handicap. I am fifty-seven years of age and though happily married and with splendid relatives I have lived a private hell as long as I can remember. I am unfortunate in having what could be called a 'pug' nose — again nothing to worry about— only it is disfigured with a purple tip which glows just like the current advertisement on the television for head-clearing lozenges. I have never been able to mix freely socially, though everywhere I worked I received excellent praise and I know that I was denied promotion because of this disfigurement. I was always supposed to be a very good public speaker but I always felt that people looked at me as if I was from outer space. My own GP is a very understanding person but I could not let myself tell even him just how I really feel about this. He made an appointment for me to see a dermatologist — a good man I suppose — but he did nothing except advise me to 'face the world' as if I was some sort of neurotic. My wife is a gem and I feel terrible for she must get tired of making excuses as to why I can't accompany her to different functions. I will travel anywhere and any fee you wish to charge you may have. Please reply and help me. Wishing you luck in your campaign to have facial disfigurement accepted by society — when you consider how society's attitude to mental illness has changed in past years I'm sure you have already achieved a great deal'.

'I read your article in the paper and I have a patient who has a congenital disfigurement below one eye and she has attended plastic surgeons and attended combined plastic surgery at dermatological clinics until she was completely fed up. I believe she would be very suitable for skin camouflage and she would be prepared to travel anywhere. *G.P.*

'I read the article 'Mark of Courage' by Joan Reeder about your work in the magazine *Woman*. I have had a scar from my ear and down my throat since I was eleven when I had tubercular glands removed. I am now in my sixties. Before I die I would like to enter a room or go into company with an unscarred neck — or at least with the illusion of one. Even now my husband has only to mention the annual dinner or some such occasion for me to be filled with dread, but you will know all these feelings. What I would like to know is where is your clinic and how do I get an appointment? I will look forward to your reply and bless you for the good work you are doing'.

'I have a problem and I would be most grateful for any advice or information you can give me. I have facial scarring over a large area but have never managed to find satisfactory cosmetics to help me. Another problem now is that such things are always so expensive. I didn't mind before as I always managed to buy what I needed; now my husband has a disease and can never work again and we are now on Invalidity Pension so I find such things too expensive. I do feel that the likes of me should be a special case but my doctors says it is not on the NHS which I think is a great pity as I cannot face going outdoors without some kind of camouflage to give me some confidence. I have heard that you worked very hard for people with problems like mine and I was so pleased to hear this as I thought our plight forgotten'.

'Could you be kind enough to arrange an appointment for this seventy-year-old woman. She has a bad port wine stain on her left cheek and of the chin and she had a skin graft carried out on the chin many years ago which is also very ugly. She is so conscious of her deformity that she has worn a scarf round the lower part of her face for the last 40 years and would be extremely grateful for your advice'. *Consultant Plastic Surgeon.*

'There is so much we want to put in this letter. Firstly we would really like to thank you for giving us hope for our little boy. He is now 19 months old, and was born with a port wine stain covering most of his body and his face. He has been into hospital seven times since he was born with convulsions and chest infections. Maybe if he hadn't been born with the port wine stain we would not feel so hurt, but as soon as he gets over one thing he has another. We have always taken him out even though we get terribly hurt every time we do. People stare, point, laugh. We try not to listen for baby's sake but hear it deep down. It is only those who have been through it who know and understand. He is our only child and we have been heartbroken more than once, but he has given us so much love and joy in so many other ways which make up for it all. Please would you let us know the procedure for an appointment'.

'I am taking the liberty of writing to you about a young Oxford undergraduate who, through an unfortunate road accident, suffered severe facial burns. I have been seeing her in this clinic because of a depressive reaction, but she has now considerably improved and is working quite well. She has had quite a lot of plastic surgery, but there is more envisaged, probably after her Oxford career finishes and in the meantime she is very sensitive about her appearance. I may say that, as a result of the plastic surgery, there is a very considerable improvement, but the scarring is still obvious. She saw your article in the *Sunday Times* and would very much appreciate it if she could possibly see you. She would be willing to come for a private consultation. I am sure that if you could manage to see her it would be most helpful to her; but she has been warned that it may be difficult to achieve a perfect cosmetic result as her scarring is still a little uneven'. *Consultant Psychiatrist.*

'I would be grateful for any help you can give me as I am badly scarred on my legs. Some years ago I consulted my doctor and he said I was too old. However. I am very conscious of the scars and try to hide them as best I can but people stare at my legs, especially on public transport. I usually stand so that I can hide them with my hand or shopping bag but this makes me so tired if I am travelling long distances'.

'I have read about your wonderful work in camouflage. My daughter, aged fourteen, has been undergoing plastic surgery on her nose and the surgeon has told us that the skin grafted on will always be a different colour from the rest of her nose and that the only remedy is expensive make-up not available on the National Health. I am therefore very interested in any information you can give me to help my daughter face the world again with confidence. She wears an ugly plaster on her nose all the time at the moment'.

'This woman suffers from socially debilitating vitiligo of the face, neck and hands. She has already been in contact with you. She recently lost her husband from cancer of the lung, has become very withdrawn and introverted, and has been keeping her own company because she is so self-conscious about her depigmentation. I should be most grateful if you could consider her as a patient for skin camouflage'. *Family Doctor.*

'I take the liberty of writing to you in the hope that you will be able to help our eighteen-year-old daughter. Some years ago whilst out with her sister she was attacked by a man with a knife, for no reason at all. He stabbed her repeatedly. Luckily, a man in a passing car intervened and a doctor was with her very quickly. How she survived is a mystery for she had been stabbed more than twenty times and had to have operations to repair internal damage. I can't praise the skill of the surgeons enough but she is dreadfully scarred and there is nothing else that they can do for her. We would be so grateful for your help in any way'.

'This patient has minimal facial blemishes but in view of an associated psychiatric disorder the inability to camouflage them effectively is proving a major disability in her life. I should be most grateful if this patient could be sent an appointment direct to attend your camouflage clinic. *Consultant Dermatologist.*

'Please accept our many thanks for all your help and making a gorgeous little boy 'matching all over everywhere' as he puts it'.

My letter is provoked by the small piece in *The Sunday Times.*
  I have suffered from the N.H.S. with my skin from about the age of 12/13 (I am now nearly 40). I went to and from my G.P. at that time and to the hospital

in Fitzroy Square to no avail and I have an acne marked face from that time.

My G.P. had absolutely no sympathy when I recently plucked up courage to ask him to refer me to a plastic surgeon or even for skin peeling treatment which I had read was helpful to acne sufferers. His reply was that the N.H.S. would not pay for any treatment at my age! Apparently if I had been 18 and my skin was affecting my marriage prospects the N.H.S. would have been prepared to help.

This of course does not help since when I was 18 if that sort of treatment had been available then I certainly was not offered it.

I have tried all my life to cover up my skin and concentrate on my hair and eyes which are reasonably good and to develop my personality but however hard you try to live with this sort of thing it does mark your mind and it is your face that other people see first of all.

I cannot afford private plastic surgery and I cannot tell you how grateful I would be if you could tell me where I could obtain advice on cosmetic camouflage.

I appreciate that my problems do not compare with those of people scarred by burns, birthmarks or accidents and, of course, limited N.H.S. resources must provide for those people first but my face (such as it is) is the only one I've got and it means a lot to me'.

'Today is my 45th birthday, and I pray to God I will never live to see my 46th birthday.

You ask to hear from persons who feel at a disadvantage as a result of their appearance. Please excuse the handwriting as I suffer from rheumatoid arthritis. I am unsightly, due to gross deformity of the hands, feet, legs and worst of all the cerebral vertebrae. I wear an orthopaedic collar. It looks and feels like a horse collar. Children stare at me in the street, my husband shuns me. Needless to say I am not asked out very often. Surgery is out of the question. I have osteoporosis — my bones would crumble if anyone knocked in nails or plates.

I am a trained nurse. I should accept this, but do I? No. Anyone with any disfigurement from any cause is at a disadvantage; society does not want to know; they will be shunned'.

3: SELF-HELP

Letter after letter each day through our letter box would tell the same, unhappy story, of alienation, of feeling cut off from other people, of disinterest in their problems, of trying to understand and come to terms with their situation, and so Peter and I decided that we would try to start a newsletter that could be a meeting place — a talking, sharing 'haven' for everyone, regardless of age or location.

We called our newsletter *Talkabout-Camouflage* and hoped that with a regular 'friend' through the letter box, no one would need to feel completely isolated or alone any more. We felt, too, that an interplay of ideas would be beneficial in every way and that many people would be helped to understand their own problems and to keep them in better perspective by reading about other people's experiences, the wisdom gained from their failures and the inspiration of their achievements.

As the months went by, we were delighted to find that readers were making friends through the pages of *Talkabout*. We found that reading of the ways in which other people had approached problems similar to their own was often the catalyst that enabled people to set down their own feelings and anxieties for the very first time. Many found great relief in being able to express their feelings, without pressure, in their own good time and uninhibited by any of the shyness that renders many inarticulate in hospital settings and secure in the knowledge that their letters and thoughts would be received with understanding. As have other caring organisations, we found that the immediacy of a letter, the thought of being straight away in direct contact, both with an individual and with a whole group of people with a common problem,

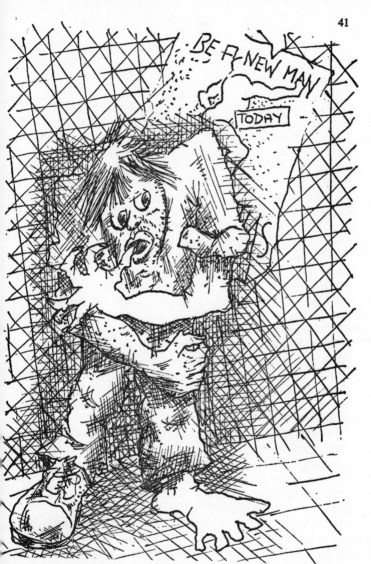

If you need a good figure to attract girls, there's no point in even dreaming.

provided an effective safety-valve and often would be the first step on the road towards a greater involvement in many other ways.

In addition there was the added benefit: to set your problems out, you must, first, identify and analyse them and when you can examine your problems quietly, honestly, patiently, you have made the first, very positive approach to the solving or containing of these same problems.

One of the nicest things that happened was the way in which so many little children took to the idea of 'Young Talkabout' with their very own special section of *Talkabout-Camouflage*. The correspondence with my younger patients is a very real, serious part of my work with them and their reaction to the newsletter was a special joy. From my own childhood experience, even when surrounded by marvellous aunts, uncles and cousins, there were lonely patches in the growing-up process and one needed lots of life-lines. If you are 'different' the idea of 'belonging' is very important and we had hoped to develop the pages of 'Young Talkabout', so that we could help younger children to find their own special friends all over the world. We sent out many thousands of copies each month, largely at our own expense, and it was warmly welcomed and requested but, at the time of writing, sadly, we have been forced to suspend publication until we can find the funds to enable us to resume printing and posting.

Encouraged by the response to, and the benefits derived from, the 'Helping Hand' of the newsletter and our growing contact with voluntary organisations, it became obvious that there would be many advantages if we could arrange informal group meetings. The first of these Self-Help Groups met at Strathclyde University, Glasgow, in October, 1974; an 'historic' occasion and the beginning of further group meetings in major centres. The development of further groups, affiliated to the voluntary services, is one of our main concerns as, in addition to the contact and supportive environment provided by group activities, the network of interest created among other members of the community assists understanding and we hope that the establishment of more Self-Help Groups, together with all our other activities, will ensure that, within the foreseeable future, people who are visually handicapped will no longer feel that they are neglected, forgotten, derided, isolated or alone.

'Every individual is unique, but our uniqueness is developed through interdependence and interaction with other unique individuals'.

Some of the people who have helped and cared: cared sufficiently to put down their thoughts and experiences to help others and try to create a kinder climate of public opinion share their courage and wisdom in the following pages . . . . .

'*Sarcoid* was a word which meant nothing to me until Sarcoidosis was diagnosed as the cause of what, up till then, I had believed to be a nose allergy. From then onwards things went from bad to worse; swelling appeared in my nose and around my eyes, unsightly lumps appeared on my cheek and arms and legs, and worst of all, the facial swelling resulted in redness which became increasingly difficult to disguise.

At this time, between hospital visits, when the doctors did all they could for me, I had phases of despair and became very depressed, despite the fact that my wedding was only a few months off. In desperation, I tried various creams, lotions and different types of make-up, hoping that they might help the condition, but all I could do was to disguise the redness, now increasing at an alarming rate, in a manner which to my mind was not very satisfactory.

Our wedding day was perfect. Miraculously, it seemed, a feeling of elation came over me, dispelling all my doubts as to whether my courage would fail me at the last minute, for previously, I had dreaded the thought of all eyes being on the bride. I may have looked the 'blushing bride', but the blush was not the sort I would have wished for. However, everyone assured me how lovely I looked, and I believed them.

Our marriage proved to be a great source of strength to me, which was fortunate as the Sarcoid was to play further havoc with my face. Despite reassurances from various doctors that the condition would go in time, I felt, in my despairing state of mind, that they were just saying this to cheer me up, for my face continued to swell, and my nose began to ulcerate, which, of course, was very distressing.

It was around this time that I had the good fortune to read about Doreen and her marvellous work and a consultation with her was arranged. Despite her expert knowledge, she had to admit that my face was in such a state that there was very little she could do at that time (although she gave me several useful tips) and she strongly advised me to seek, via my doctor, the help of a leading consultant, noted for his work in this particular field. I decided immediately to take her advice and I can now state that this was the turning point of my life.

After undergoing tests, I was given drugs to check the swelling, and already I looked a different person. Doreen had literally saved my face. I continued to travel to London for a little over twelve months, and was eventually transferred to an excellent local skin specialist who still supervises my treatment.

Unfortunately, in the early days of the condition, (before Sarcoid was diagnosed) I had had an experimental operation on my nose, and also, later on, I had several injections in my nose. Once the swelling had subsided, my nose assumed a state of disfigurement, and there is no question of plastic surgery at the moment, as the condition is still active, although controlled. The redness is no longer a problem, thanks to the excellent selection of foundations now on the market, but the stigma of my disfigured nose remains. As with any abnormality, it is extremely difficult to accept that one 'looks different' and it was this aspect of the disease with which I found hardest to cope.

However, I can now say that I have at last managed to come to terms with it; something which at one time I wouldn't have thought possible. I have found that by adapting my life style to the condition I am much happier and have even found peace of mind.

For instance, I try to keep myself occupied all the time, especially mentally, for when one's mind is occupied, there is no time to brood over or worry about one's appearance. Naturally, I do not like crowds, but then I have never done, and I automatically try to avoid them, but on the occasions when it is necessary to mix with them, especially strangers, I dress in my most striking and trendy clothes, and wear plenty of eye make-up. This gives me a feeling of confidence, which otherwise I would lack. A smile goes a long way too. It is surprising how people will ignore imperfections, when greeted by a cheerful, smiling face.

I feel happiest and most at ease when with my family (including my in-laws) and close friends for I am fortunate to be surrounded by people who apparently see only the inner person and like me for what I am, as opposed to what I look like. I truly count my blessings and believe that life 'balances up'.

I always try and maintain a sense of humour over my condition. It is surprising how this can help. Once I had accepted it (by far the most difficult part) and eventually managed to raise the odd smile, I considered I was at least half way to overcoming the psychological effects. I often joke about having 'a new nose' (which I hope I shall have one day) as if they were advertised in the 'Articles for Sale' columns.

Seriously, though, I look forward to that day when the condition will have disappeared. I have had a lot of heartbreak because of this strange disease, but it has also brought me much happiness, for through it, I have discovered real contentment with the simple things of life, and a peace of mind I might otherwise never have known. Also I shall never take anything, especially my health, for granted again.

For these reasons, the experience has not been a wasted one. I do hope, sincerely, that my story may bring a slight ray of hope to anyone who feels full of despair, as I once did, and encourage others not to give up in the long struggle to regain one's confidence.

If any readers who have had similar experiences to those I have mentioned would care to write to me, I shall be only too pleased to reply, for I know too well the terrible feeling of isolation which accompanies any sort of facial disfigurement. How often I have wished to have someone to confide in who really understands through personal experience what you are going through.

My best wishes to all readers of *Talkabout Camouflage* and congratulations to all who help to produce it. May this enterprising newsletter achieve all the success which it deserves'.

'I feel I must write to you with regard to the letter of Mrs M. King in your February issue of *Talkabout*.

When my husband and I read Mrs King's letter it was like reading our own past story. Our daughter, Maria, is now 9 years of age and only recently did we decide to acquire a cover cream.

Together with a Doctor friend of ours we discussed, before Maria started school, whether or not to cover up the port wine stain which covers her right cheek, part eyelid and disappears into the hair. We finally decided not to because of the question: 'What will Maria do if ever found without her cosmetics on?' We decided this would be more hurtful than leaving her birthmark uncovered.

We have never wrapped the fact up that her birthmark is there. We refer to it by name. Maria herself will tell you that it will never go and that the only thing she can do is cover it up with make-up. I feel so strongly that you must from the beginning tell the truth; it certainly has helped and worked with Maria. By accepting the truth the child gains the confidence needed to face others who are more fortunate and by the same token realise how lucky they are when seeing others less fortunate than themselves, i.e. Spastics, etc.

The time will come, Mrs King, when your daughter will ask you to take her birthmark away; this I found so upsetting but I still explained the truth to her and then went into the bathroom for a good cry.

Our daughter is a really lovely child, her personality alone will get her far. She has a great compassion for a child of nine. She has the ability to dance well and this too has given her confidence.

When the Lord gave Maria a birthmark He also gave her something else extra special as I'm sure He did Mrs King's daughter'.

'After twelve years of childless marriage, my husband and I were so thrilled when we learned we were going to have our first baby. Like all parents we began to plan, and prepare only the best for our child, never thinking for a minute that anything could happen at the birth.

Our life seemed to shatter when our little girl was born with a birth mark over her face. I think we cried till we couldn't cry any more. Friends tried to help us by saying the mark would fade, and that Doctors would be able to do something about it, but they, the Doctors, seemed to hurt us more when we heard them refer to it as 'The Port Wine Stain'.

We went to see Doctors and Specialists with our hopes built up that they would be able to help our little girl, each time coming home with the same story — that she would always have the mark on her face as nothing could be done about it.

One Doctor was sorry that no one in the medical profession had ever done anything about the birth-mark, and another told us to get it into our heads that our child was as good as the next. We know that our little girl is as good, if not better, in our eyes, but how it hurts us when we are out in the streets or shops or buses and can see people's reactions to our child. They hurt us more, as our little girl is only two years old, and doesn't understand yet. Some people look with sadness and sorrow; others can be very cruel and so unkind in what they say and in the way they stare at our child.

All our hopes were shattered until I read an article in a magazine about Mrs Trust.

I wrote to the Editor who put me in touch with her. We were so filled up with nerves when we took our little girl to the Western Infirmary to see if she could do anything for her as this was to be our last resort. What a lovely person, and someone who really shared our little girl's problem, as well as ours, and who has given us hope by being able to help our child.

I am quite sure that some day we will all be able to go out, just like anyone else, and not have the thought of people staring at us and with our child feeling just like any other little child.

I can only hope, Mrs Trust, that you get the support to carry out the wonderful work that you are doing.

If anyone has a child with this problem and feels as thought they just can't face it, I will be only too willing to help them . . . . '

'As one who is very interested in the work you are trying to achieve, may I congratulate you on the way your first Glasgow Group meeting was conducted.

It has been said 'That a journey of one thousand miles begins with the first step' and I believe that you and your group started on that road, on the 5th September, in the University of Strathclyde.

The points raised and ground covered must augur well for the future well-being of the groups. To see and meet such a large turn-out on so wet and miserable an evening makes one feel that you are heading in the right direction.

I send both you and the groups my best wishes for continued success, and hope that through caring and sharing with each other you shall continue going from strength to strength'.

'As the ambulance took me and my two-day-old daughter from the maternity unit home to my waiting husband and three-year-old son, the sun shone down on a lovely warm May morning, and no one in the world could have been happier than I.

Only ten days later, however, a small cloud had started to arise on our horizon, for as the midwife bathed my baby, I noticed what I thought to be a tiny fingernail scratch on the lower lid of her left eye, which I assumed she had inflicted on herself. Several days passed in which it appeared to have made no progress in healing, and if anything, had increased just a fraction in size. On attending Clinic, the Welfare Officer confirmed that this mark was a naevus growing on my small daughter's eyelid, and I was referred to a Specialist at my local hospital. After examination, he advised me that this was destined to get larger over the next six months and, shatteringly, there was nothing they could do but to let it take its course.

To have to sit back and watch a dark-red-erased crescent growing bigger and bigger on the face of a little girl is a truly dreadful experience, and even although I was assured by my doctor that probably after six months it would stop growing and then eventually start to diminish and fade, which would perhaps take up to a period of seven years, I was not totally convinced, for as yet, at this moment of time, it was worsening. We could only hope and pray that medical knowledge would prove correct.

We are one of the few lucky ones, whose hopes over the last seven years have been turned to joy, as very, very gradually and month by month nature has slowly healed this ugly mark, and I doubt very much whether anyone would even notice a slight discolouration, which is, at present, all that remains, without having it pointed out.

Our experience of once having to face up to the possibility of such a scar marring our daughter for life, has given us a special understanding towards those whose disfigurement is of a permanent nature, as I have known the anguish of the attention being 'different' brings, being only thankful it was us, her parents, and not our child, who was completely un-aware of the reason or the interest she caused. How comforting it would have been to have known in the earlier years of someone like Doreen Trust who, when nothing can be done medically, has opened a door offering help by the camouflaging of such unsightly blemishes. Learning of her courageous efforts to establish clinics in this field, she has my deepest admiration, and I would very much like to extend my hand to help such a wonderful person in any way I can in my own part of the country'.

'Many years ago now, I became the victim of a rather silly, though very dangerous, prank. I was, I remember, about fourteen years of age and at the very impression-able, and rather painful stage of being a teenager.

I did know (just about) that girls, for example, did exist and I also knew that I had to be accepted as one of the group irrespective of my own personal feelings or beliefs for, at this age, one thinks that unless you are with, or seen with a social group of similarly-minded teenagers, then there must, of course, be some-thing wrong with you.

During this era of bravado and attention-seeking, which I must stress as being quite normal behaviour, myself and two other friends, having just recently procured the devilish device of a shotgun, decided that it would be advantageous to our boyish egoes to brandish the said devilish device upon any conceivable thing that may show promise, i.e. runs, crawls or flies.

However, after a very fruitless 'sport' we eventually decided to rest. Boys will be boys, or so we are led to believe and one of our party started to play with this hardly untouched shotgun and, yes, you guessed, it went off in my face.

The rest of this tale is rather boring perhaps because many similar occurrences happen every day without fail. The important thing to me, and to the many other people in a similar position, is what happens *after* all the hospital care, tests, operations, etc. are finished with and when you eventually realise that you may not be, perhaps, just as handsome or pretty as you may have been before, and when people, even so-called friends, in your absence, describe you, not by your name, but by that particular mark, burn, scar or whatever on your face, arms, legs or wherever you may have it. So you may consider that your pride is hurt and that your ego is somewhat depleted and this is now the problem that you have to face. As far as I know, there is no miraculous cure to make you quite so wholesome as before, but this does not mean to say that there is nothing you can do. For those of you like myself, by all means try camouflage as an aid in this effort to build up from this feeling of having a broken or shaken ego but, please, do not rely wholly upon it. Use the camouflage for as long as you find it necessary, then leave it off for a while and see if your feelings of inadequacy are still quite so strong as they may have been previously. I sincerely hope not! '

'My son was born on 1st July, 1964. A mongol child. This meant absolutely nothing to my husband or myself. Like most people we knew that mentally and physically handicapped people are different but never gave a thought to what this might mean until we were personally involved.

The Paediatrician concerned with our son said that he would defy any lay person to tell that the child was different for at least his first year. The following summer when it became apparent that our son could not sit unaided, the comments started. One woman told me that she had known since he was born that something was wrong and that perhaps I should find out if he was blind, as well as retarded.

As our son grew older the stares were more obvious.

It would have been more acceptable to my husband and myself if they had asked outright what was wrong. We had more than our fair share of stares because we treated our son as normally as possible and did not hide him away. If we went shopping, he came too. If we had lunch in a restaurant, so did he. Sometimes a meal was a slow process but he had to learn and it kept us together as a family.

When it became known generally, that our son was a mongol, numerous people over the years have looked at him and told me he looked all right and that he will grow out of it. No amount of elementary explaining will change their minds. They may mean to be kind, but, once a parent has faced facts about their child, then these 'kindnesses' only annoy and exasperate.

When our son was nearly three, we had a second son (this one normal; if such a thing as 'normal' exists). We, ourselves, had fears that our son might not like the new baby and be harmful towards him, but waited to see. Needless to say, relatives started saying that if our son harmed the new baby he would have to go into a home and so on, but from the day the baby arrived, our son has played his part very well. The 'baby' now towers over his brother and protects him but his brother knows that he is the elder of the two and says so with great glee.

Our eldest son is now twelve years old and I know that he looks different and acts differently from other boys his age, but if only the world at large would accept him as he wants them to we might all be happier.

These seem like minor irritations now, when I am sitting here writing some of this down but at the time they were monumental obstacles — or maybe I have mellowed a lot!

'Frequently I have a migraine headache. A number of years ago I wrote a passionate article pleading for understanding. It was never sent to any publisher, but it achieved its purpose . . . it wrote itself out of my system. Little did I know what lay ahead. A facial condition which developed eight years ago caused me great anxiety. Two plastic surgery operations were technically successfully, but the condition infiltrated fairly rapidly and left not only bright red skin but a mis-shapen nose.

Well meaning people, who are only being kind, with remarks like 'It doesn't show', or 'I didn't even notice', do not really help. You know that it does show . . . goodness knows you look at it often enough. Along with this stage and its resulting depression, comes despair, disbelief, dejection, and a deterioration of former spirits. Family and friends you may have, but this as I remember it, is the fearful and frightening stage of being alone. At this point practical help and understanding are needed, not sympathy. But where do we get this special kind of help?

In common with many others, I did not know where to go, and that leaves the choice of psychiatrist or pills or nothing. It's here that you begin to win or lose. Week after week I tried new creams, thicker creams, darker creams, anything and everything which I hoped would make me look and feel normal. With each disappointment part of you dies, and you wonder how much longer you can go on. Anguish, anger, moods, temper and finally the giving-in follow. Truly I felt that life held nothing for me, and yet when I look back, the normal chores of cleaning, washing, cooking, gardening and caring for the family continued, and so I suppose that somewhere there must have been a guiding hand.

Two brilliant and dedicated men, nearing the ends of their respective tethers, along with myself, pointed me in yet another direction. One cold February morning found me heading towards the Western Infirmary in Glasgow, with a newly acquired crust, a shield against anything which may hurt or disappoint. I sat waiting to see 'the make-up lady' with head down, now my normal posture.

Those of you who have had the wonderful experience of spending time with Doreen will most certainly not need me to remind them or tell them what happens, but suffice to say that I walked out with head held high and my normal quest for cleanliness was overlooked. I didn't wash for two days.

The story doesn't end there, we all know that. There are still days of anguish and despair. Being a 'patchwork person' automatically makes one feel different. I know that I will never look normal but ninety per cent of the time I feel normal and I hope, behave in a normal way.

My story is no different from many others, but I hope that by telling it I may encourage other non-writers to put pen to paper. Somehow it does put everything in its proper perspective when you write it down.

I will be so pleased to meet anyone in this area who has a similar problem. I personally believe that it would have been helpful to me to talk with a non-friend, non-family at certain points.

I hope that you, Doreen, will be able to achieve all that you wish — which, knowing you, will all be for others. Thank you for helping to give me back my life, which after all is for living'.

'This is a page devoted entirely to fashion — I do not mean the type one sees in all the glossies, I mean the day to day sort. Fashion is purely a state of mind, by this I mean knowing particular fashions that suit your own individual self and personality. For example, I know a lady with 50″ hips and she is one of the smartest people I know. This probably sounds far fetched but when I say her clothes actually fit well all over, even her shopping coat, this is the first obstacle to be overcome. We have all at some time had a badly fitting article in which we feel frumps, but we have also had a favourite dress which we know suits us perfectly and feels right each time it is worn. Think of the things in which you feel your best — our biggest enemy is liking something in which we look hideous. Take this same lady, she only wears soft styles. By this I mean some straight skirts, but also 'A' line and soft bias cuts which means it clings gently on the hips and swings out slightly at the hemline. Some years ago I taught dressmaking at a school with 12-15 year-old girls, and the largest girl I had longed to wear gathered skirts so much so that one day she became quite aggressive because other girls in the class were making gathered dresses, so I said she could make one —of course I was certain it could be taken to pieces again and re-used. She made up a skirt, put it on and thought she looked 'the cat's whiskers', even though the rest of the class told her the truth. That week-end she wore it to the youth club and accepted all the jeers,

telling everyone else they were jealous. This went on
for a couple of weeks, then one day she came to
class and said, 'Miss, can I undo this skirt and make
it into a style that suits me?' Of course, it was a
little different for this girl as she was only 15 and
could afford to make mistakes. It is up to us to
know our particular problem, do all we can about it,
and if there is nothing further we can do, then accept
it and dress *for it* and not *against it*.

The question of proper fitting clothes always causes
some consternation as people say they have to put
up with what they can buy at the shops. This, of course,
is true and the Head of Department at the Art College
I attended openly admitted to me one day that this
country has not got enough good designers for larger
women, 'all the kids want to design for the kids',
she said. So I can only say, buy an article which fits
on the bust, as the shoulders and sleeves are the most
difficult to alter. The skirt does not present such
problems. I do know that all over the British Isles
there are these marvellous little dressmakers, just around
the corner, and the ones I know are always the sort
that will put themselves out to help an unfortunate
rather than the flighty little miss who wants to be
the belle of the ball. But when buying clothes from a
shop do not be fobbed off by 'Madam it suits you
beautifully'. I have had some of this myself and know
very well that it looks hideous. If you are the sort of
person who does not like to walk out of a shop without
buying, and the British female has this reputation,
then tell the assistant you will have to bring back
your husband, mother or sister to see it before you
can buy it. Please do not think I am trying to encourage
you to tell lies, but I have seen some very sad cases
of poor old ladies being talked into something when
it was only too obvious it did not suit them. But, I am
not suggesting for one minute that all our sales-ladies
are like this. Far from it, I have also come across
some extremely honest and fair ones who tell you the
whole truth. All I am trying to say is that we need to
be on our guard a little more than the next person
because of a hidden disability.

Also, when I was teaching, I came across an alarming
number of girls who used to tell me they could not
sew and hated it. So I would start with a simple skirt

and can tell you that by the end of two terms these same girls were making quite elaborate styles, so much so, that whilst I was there, I put on two fashion shows and the audience were quite taken aback to see the sort of clothes the girls had made themselves. So it might be worthwhile doing a short course, say September to May, at your local evening class, and some do have classes during the day also. But do not begin with a complicated style, rather start with a very simple cut and try to pick up as many tips as possible. These can all be taken from books, I know, but it is much simpler to grasp it, if somebody actually shows you how to do it at first hand.

I would like you to send me your particular query and any fashion problem you may have. I will endeavour to answer as many as possible, with a few suggestions on how to camouflage your particular fashion problem. I do believe that almost everything can be made obscure. I do know personally of the embarrassment and even shame one feels when we know we are not like other people we see every day and the fact that everybody tells us we are stupid because others do not see our faults is no help whatsoever. So if we can cover up our disability then we do so, but also, at the same time, we must make all we can of the good assets we have. We all have some good point although I know that at times this is hard to believe.

'But to look on the bright side, there appears to be a definite awakening of interest in the difficulties faced by the facially disfigured. I've come to believe more and more that the correct approach is an aggressive attacking one. Shout it out loud and clear at the 'normals' that *they* should be shamed of their prejudices, not the disfigured of their faces!

All persecuted and ostracised minorities, who have successfully broken through the barriers have done so by militant action. Not by pleading humbly to be permitted to exist at their oppressors' pleasure. It's up to us to make discrimination, socially and in employment, on grounds of physical disfigurement as unacceptable in a so-called enlightened society, as certain other forms of discrimination have become. I've already done my best to build up a little 'cell' of sympathisers in my own club — quite amusing at times to watch some 'intellectual' engaged in a mental wrestling match between his natural instincts and his fashionable social conscience.

However, it's still partly up to us; we must be prepared to make allowance for the primitive fear all people have of things that are different (a perfectly rational and reasonable caution in many contexts) and above all, show ourselves, although disfigured, to be sane, mentally normal and rational human beings. All too often, like a certain type of coloured man who is always seeing racial discrimination where it does not exist, many of our people have become hypersensitive, and consequently *are* shunned, not necessarily because of their appearance but on account of their embarrassing character distortions and aggressions. I can see this only too well in myself: I can relax much better in company now, and not care whether I'm rejected or accepted by people when I first meet them — I am getting big-headed and arrogant enough these days to consider it's their loss!

4: SOME CASE HISTORIES

Mr T.E.

A family recluse will affect the stability and prosperity of the whole family.

This man had suffered from *chronic discoid lupus erthematosus* of the face and scalp which was inactive but which had left extensive and disfiguring scarring. Such was the embarrassment caused by his appearance both to himself and to his family, that he had retired and led the life of a recluse. He had totally lost interest in himself and even refused to wear his false teeth as he felt that 'nothing mattered anymore'. After a number of sessions at the Skin Camouflage Clinic he was fully competent in the application of a basic covering paste and three skin colourants and could do this, unaided in some ten minutes. It would have been possible to construct, from his own hair, a small prosthesis to fill in a badly distorted eyebrow line and this would have added to the improvement and from my own point of view I would have preferred so to do. Mr T.E. however, felt that the wearing of any such aid would bother him and was so pleased with his altered appearance that the distortion no longer bothered him and, therefore, this final improvement was not effected.

Because of the extensive damage to the skin surface, the end result in such cases is usually far from perfect but it can lessen the initial impact so greatly that the patient feels once more able to face up to the world, instead of cringeing from its cruel reactions. Mr T.E felt so greatly encouraged that, at his last session with me he announced that he was going straight back home to put his false teeth in to complete his new appearance and outlook! Within a very short time he returned to an active

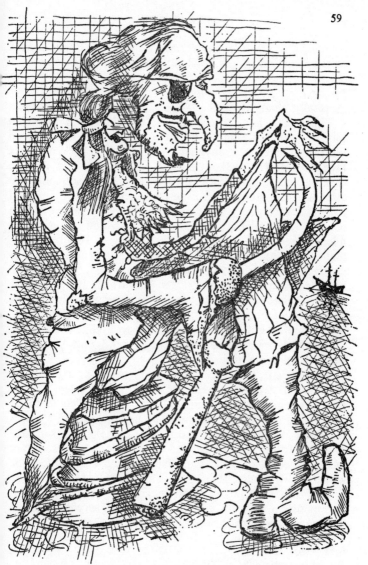

Sometimes the pressures can make you act the part you look.

working life, with obvious material and emotional benefit to the function of the total family unit.

Mr M.L.: *aged twenty-one.*
A totally changed outlook, life style and career prospect.

This youth has an extensive port wine stain involving most of the left side of his face and neck which caused him so much embarrassment that he felt he could not face people. He walked around with a stooping posture tucking the affected side of his face into his chest. He also suffered from severe *psoriasis.* When he emerged from his first period of camouflage care his alteration in bearing was dramatic. He stood upright, had a more confident aspect and was obviously overjoyed. Frequent contacts throughout the next two years established a totally changed outlook which has persisted. His *psoriasis* has has cleared and he now has a job, which he previously had not. The change, not only in appearance but in bearing and social composure and confidence was such that when, some time later he accompanied me to a clinical meeting, his general practitioner who was present, and knew him well, failed to recognise him.

At a recent group meeting, some seven or eight years after my first contact with Mr M.L., he attended, accompanied by his mother who said that she had come to be able to thank me in person for the miraculous changes that had occurred as a result of the help her son had received from my clinics and that this had altered, not only her son's outlook, but had affected and united the whole family group.

This now very popular and successful young man holds a responsible position within the hospital services and, in his spare time, leads a flourishing pop group.

Mrs V.M.
Breathing space to re-adjust.

This lady is the wife of a very senior academic in one

of our premier universities and as such, led an extremely active social life. The development of *lupus pernio of Hutchinson* with a particularly deep erthrocyanotic tint forced a drastic curtailment of her activities and led to a deeply depressive state when topical and intralesional steroid had no effect. Skin Camouflage assistance proved satisfactory and the understanding and unhurried contact at a series of clinic sessions gave this eminently courageous and intelligent woman essential 'breathing space' in which to regain her equilibrium and perspective, adjust and re-assemble her attitudes and muster the confidence to resume her social life and many family commitments.

Miss M.C.K.: aged forty-three years.
Death of identity and the concomitant threat to livelihood and career advancement.

This patient developed *lupus vulgaris* at the age of three years which, despite lengthy treatment had left her with extensive facial scarring. Her personality gradually deteriorated until she had to seek psychiatric aid, which helped. Eventually, she was referred to the Skin Camouflage Clinic and the combination of encouragement, general advice about dress, make-up, and the handling of difficult social problems resulting from her appearance, together with the suggested camouflage techniques has resulted in a striking improvement to her appearance and morale. She can now make herself look attractive and at last has been able to hold down a job for longer than a month. She feels that referral to the Skin Camouflage Clinic was the turning point in her life.

I have selected the above case history for a very special reason. After an interim period of some seven or eight years, this patient now, typically and predictably, feels the need to return for further advice and guidance. This happens to most patients, as age, changing circumstances and needs require that they should modify their appearance;

or as skin deterioration in skin diseases, or the unexpected side effects of drugs prescribed as part of the patient's treatment demand further adaption. Sometimes an unexpected unkind comment about their face, catches them off-guard and coincides with an upsurge of the unnatural fear (felt by so many) of the quite natural ageing processes which exacerbates this latter condition and leads to a sudden erosion of both present confidence and future hope.

This very real fear cannot lightly be dismissed as this possible death of identity will be felt as a threat to livelihood and career advancement by those many disfigured people who have spent most of their lives hidden under a mask of heavy make-up. It is vitally important that contact, help and support, when needed are readily forthcoming in such cases.

An unusual consultation.

The patient was 5ft 3ins and rather plump (10st 6lb). Her hair was a bleached blonde, her eyes dark brown and her skin sallow, coarsely textured and with residual acne vulgaris pitting. She had a history of many problems and felt that her face had been a socially crippling influence for almost as long as she could remember. She had an aversion to make-up and felt that it made her look older and 'made-up'.

When this patient came to see us she was wearing a strong red lipstick and had heavily lined and darkened eyebrows. She was wearing an ice-blue two-piece suit with a matching open-necked, heavy lace blouse; the jacket of the suit flared from the waist and her skirt length was just above the knee. Her appearance, as she later agreed, was an unfortunate assemblage of unbalances because these had been done without thought of the total and finished result.

The Art Consultant and I combined our opinions, analysed and discussed these with the patient and then all agreed on an appropriate and positive course of action.

Basic revision. We suggested a simplification of the elaborate night-time ritual involving a whole array of largely unnecessary, rejuvenating preparations and pointed out that it was much better to follow a simple, basic routine *every* night than a complicated ritual twice weekly. We obtained an undertaking from the patient that she would follow this simple routine every night and morning for the next three weeks — a short and feasible time, but sufficient to effect an improvement and so encourage a further three weeks' effort — by which time, we hoped, it would have become habitual.

We recommended an alternating programme of preparations selected from the range of those specified for our patient as we have found our own 'rhythmic' approach to be psychologically attractive as well as beneficial in its more obvious effects.

a rosemary/vegetable soap for the highly perfumed super-fatted one in use.

b a simple lotion, to be made freshly every other day, in place of the over-strong, degreasing astringent.

Colour balance and co-ordination. We had decided that the colour 'common denominator' with which we could co-ordinate our subject in total would be in the darker golden browns and proceeded accordingly.

In view of the patient's dislike of make-up we decided that it would be of little assistance to devise ways of infilling the more obvious acne pittings and instead concentrated on the use of a minimum amount of colour, strategically positioned, so as to:

a enliven the face without making it appear artificial and

b lift the eye to the heart-shaped unflawed area of cheek-bone, temple and eye orbit

after which we would 'scumble' the entire face.

The patient had had her hair dyed blonde in an attempt to conceal grey hairs and did not wish to revert to her natural mid-brown/grey mixture, but agreed with us that the tone should be softened when she had her next tinting session.

Meantime, we used temporarily a powder to tone down the hair and illustrate the intended effect. We lightened the eyebrows, pencilling in individual lines, to the natural direction of brow growth with two different colours of eye-brow pencil and introduced some brown eye tones to balance the very dark eyes which had previously stood out of her face looking hard and almost black.

After some trial and error we found a combination of items which satisfied all our requirements: agreed that this was a colour-balanced and pleasing total improvement; that the preparations employed to effect this were both safe and suitable; and that it was feasible in every respect so that the patient could quickly and easily duplicate the whole process without further outside assistance.

The total look.   By measuring our patient's appearance 'pros' and 'cons' against the basic rules of colour balance and composition, then modifying and re-arranging these within our original concept of her appearance, we had created an elegant and attractive face, using a great deal of art and a very little make-up. We had an enthusiastic and delighted patient and so we continued. We elongated the nail shape, changing the colour of her nail enamel and pointed out that her excess of jewellery and chunky dress rings detracted from, rather than enhanced, her rather attractive hands; they were removed willingly.

We then discussed colour and body line and the Art Consultant illustrated various aspects of this as it affected our patient. We selected from our files a calf-length dress in brown and beige and illustrated how this would slender-ise and lengthen her body line, pointing out that the darker basic colours would also help to shade a too plump and decidedly ageing throat line. As a final touch we showed how the illusion of further elongation could be achieved by the selection of harmonising shoes and stockings. The picture that emerged was that of an integrated, graceful and elegant looking woman.

We invited the patient's husband in to comment and become involved so that he would encourage his wife. The state of this patient's skin had often caused social events to be missed by both husband and wife and had been a source of distress to them both for many years despite the husband's assurances that it didn't matter. Surprisingly, many wives or husbands will talk about the problem but not about their feelings, and it can often clear the air and create a new bond of understanding between them to talk together to us as they can do so without restraint or fear of appearing foolish. There is an additional advantage in that an approving husband involvement and the renewal of interest and awareness of 'the wife' as a person, is often just the little 'extra' needed to set off a whole chain reaction of re-appraisals and a more positive approach to problems in many other spheres, sometimes with surprisingly beneficial results to the whole family unit . . . A 'mum' who is pleased with herself, her accomplishments, and her life is a joy to all!

E

5: ONLY SKIN DEEP

Basic skin information

A knowledge of the basic anatomy and physiology of the skin is a prerequisite to any sensible and effective programme of skin maintenance and skin camouflage. So what are the things to keep in mind?

Part of the body's protection is in its architecture and the materials of which it is made; from the marvellous functional architecture of the human skeleton to its remarkable, self-protecting, self-repairing outer covering — the skin. It is sometimes forgotten that the skin does more than 'keep the rest of us in', that it is, in fact, the largest organ of the body, and comprises roughly 16% of the total body weight. It also contains between 25% and 40% of the body's extra-cellular fluid and is an important storage organ of water, most of which is contained in the **dermis.** Our skin is suited to our own environment and comes in all textures and colours but, unlike the skin of whales and other aquatic mammals whose outer covering is structured to provide an effective water barrier, it is not absolutely air-tight or water-tight. One of the reasons that human cross channel swimmers have to grease themselves heavily is to reduce percutaneous water absorption. A body submerged in water for any length of time would become oedematous and look bloated; a process we have probably all experienced and observed in the strange 'crinkling' of our fingers if we have had our hands in water for even quite short periods. This 'skin drinking' is called hydration and it is balanced, like every other process in a normal healthy body, by our being, also, in a constant state of 'evaporation'. It has been estimated that, in a temperate

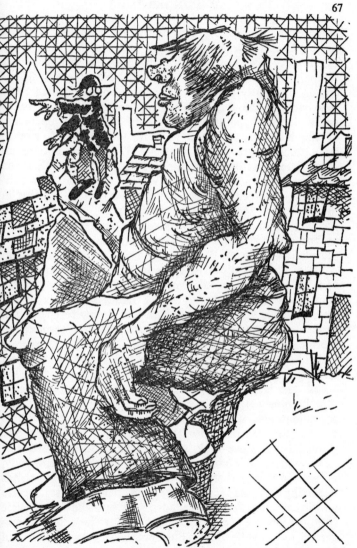

Being big doesn't mean I'm clumsy or violent. I love beautiful delicate things.

climate, in comfortable conditions, a male adult will lose
some 120 ml of water per square metre of his skin, every
24 hours, via his skin's transepidermal route. Body
temperature is thermostatically controlled at about 37° C
and is constantly monitored by nerve endings which relay
this back to the thermoregulatory centre near the sweat
centre in the hypothalamus, and through the temperature
of the blood as it passes near the mid-brain. A rise in
body temperature of above some 37° C will initiate an
immediate sweating response irrespective of whether the
increase is from muscular activity or a rise in skin temperature, whereas the skin has a lower sweating point in
the region of 34° C. It is a reminder of man's frailty to
recall that the astronauts were supplied with suits in-
corporating a system of water cooled pipes so as to prevent
thermal sweating on their awe-inspiring trips to the moon.

There are two different types of sweat glands and some
2½-3 million small sweat glands in the human body, these
being especially numerous on the hands and soles of the
feet. In three groupings — trunk and limbs, forehead and
axillae and the palmer and plantar which respond to
thermoregulatory or emotional stimuli, or both, and secrete
a slightly acid fluid which probably has an inhibitory effect
on any harmful skin bacteria, via ducts through the skin
pores. The large sweat glands of the axillae and urogenital
skin become active at adolescence, appear to be hormone
dependent and it is this apocrine sweat secretion which
exudes the familiar 'sweaty' smell. Modified apocrine
glands also produce milk, and the wax of the external ear.

The sebaceous glands are also distributed over the body,
except on the palms and soles with the largest glands
occurring on the scalp, face and back. These secrete
an oily, waste substance called sebum into the hair follicle
from which they originally develop as flask-shaped epidermal outgrowths. The sebum coats the growing hair and
permeates into the superficial cells of the horny layer, where
it helps to keep the skin supple and water-proofed.

Repeated degreasing of the skin makes it sensitive and susceptible to irritants and although about 50% is replaced within about an hour by the continual secretion of the sebaceous gland it is easy to forget and over-use strong chemicals and degreasers; hence all those housework hands. Sebum production is much lower in pre-adolescent children and so a child's skin will 'chap' easily. Lanolin and wool fat which we find in many of our ointments and cosmetics is, in fact the sebaceous secretion of sheep.

Although we can define skin structure it is important to remember that the skin is not a collection of separate parts but interdependent layers combined in a functional whole, reflecting the health of, and nourished by, the body it covers and in a constant state of activity.

The human skin is divided into two different, interlocking and mutually dependent layers. The epidermis or visible surface, derived, along with the nervous system, from that part of the basic body cell, the embryonic ectoderm, is made up of numerous cells, varying in shape and substance and arranged in four or five 'pavement' layers in which the progression towards formation of the outer, surface cell, the protein keratin takes place.

The outer layer of the epidermis is constantly being worn away and replaced by the new cells formed from mitotic division in the lowest or basal layer. As the new cells ascend they undergo a series of changes in shape and substance. Granules form in them and finally they die, lose their outline and form a continuous protective sheet of keratin.

Normally the proliferation of new cells exactly balances the shedding of dead cells from the skin's surface so that the thickness of the epidermis remains constant and radioactive labelling methods have made it possible to assess that it takes some twenty-seven days for a cell from the lowest, basal layer to reach the outer layer. This varies considerably in various abnormal skin conditions and in *psoriasis* for example, the 'turnover' time is estimated to be some eight times faster than this average.

The thickness of the epidermis is dependent upon cell size and the number of cell layers which forms the structure, one of the thinnest areas is the face, and the thickest the palms and soles, where the palmer and plantar epidermis has a prominent granular layer and above this develops a narrow, and extra, layer of partly keratinised cells, called the *stratum lucidum*. When we consider our environment, in which almost everything we encounter is hard, sharper and heavier than our own soft skins we appreciate the need for the little extra 'toughness' of hands nd feet although it is interesting to note in passing that the normal human epidermis is much thicker than that of the crocodile. Happily for us, there is a great difference between us, in the thickness of the outer keratin layer each develops! The cellular layers of the epidermis are supported and nourished from the underlying, interlocking fibrous connective tissue gel of the dermis, which can be divided into the top part or superficial dermis and the lower level the deep dermis. The dermal layer acts as a framework for the blood vessels, nerves, lymphatics, hair follicles, sebaceous glands, sweat glands, arrecter pili (goose pimpley), muscles, papillae and a variety of cells derived from the mesoderm. The most numerous of these latter being the fibroblasts which synthesise collagen and, in smaller amounts, elastin and deposit them outside the cells with the result that the dermal cells become widely separated from each other as they develop.

Subcutaneous tissue or hypodermal adipose tissue is a layer of fat laden cells immediately below the dermis and contains some 60% of the store of body fat. This fatty layer has vital nutritional, thermal and protective functions as well as giving smoothness and contour to the body. It varies in thickness, according to the age, sex and general health of the person but women, normally, will have a thicker layer of fatty tissue than men, the distribution of this being determined by the endocrine glands.

The skin and hair are capable of striking variations in colour both transient and permanent and discussion of the many factors involved — some areas of which are still controversial and undetermined is beyond the scope of this present book.

The characteristic tint of the skin is genetically determined, as is the inherited biochemical 'blocks' of the congenital albino, whose skin is devoid of colour. Beyond this, the colour of the skin is due to a combination of three things. First the blood supply, we can go white with fear, blue with cold, red with anger, due to the closure, stasis or increase of the blood flow and secondly, the natural yellowish 'colour' of the dermis and epidermal cells — the natural skin colour. In addition to these two things there is a yellowish-brown pigment called melanin which is synthesised in special cells known as melanocytes lying in the basal layer of the epidermis.

A chemically slightly different type of melanin is largely responsible for the hair pigmentation that produces, amongst other of nature's marvels, the leopard's spots and the stripes of the zebra and although it also gives us our yellow, red, black and browns, if we want stripes in our hair we have to get them from a bottle of hair dye.

The sun is indispensable and although many of its rays could be harmful they are mostly absorbed in the outer atmosphere. Wave lengths of around 300 nanometres in the Ultra Violet Radiation spectrum with a fatty substance present in sebum can produce Vitamin D in the skin. Apart from this, uncontrolled UVR exposure is deleterious and ageing, although it does, indeed, feel nice. The skin reacts to the stimulus of sunlight and increases its tolerance to further exposure (one of the reasons that dermatologists advocate a gradually lengthening programme of 'sunbathing') by the production of the pigment melanin, and with a thickening of the horny, outer keratin layer. Keratin is a most unreactive protein and together with the melanin screens, absorbs and scatters the sunburning UVR. The production of melanin in coloured skins is continuous and is under genetic control whereas a 'natural' tan in the Caucasian skin is acquired through stimulation of melanin formation. Sunlight is often the stimulus that produces this although a number of diseases can also increase skin pigmentation showing 'a healthy tan' to be a somewhat meaningless phrase. Excessive sunlight is thought to be responsible for the very high incidence of a certain type of skin cancer, in Caucasian skins, in Australia, South Africa and the hotter parts of the United States; our intemperate climate has many consolations.

Since it is a complex organ, it is not surprising that the skin has several functions and when we know a little more about the structure of the skin and the nature of its functions we are better able to assist rather than impede these functions and better equipped to form our own opinion of creams and treatments that promise 'instant' beauty, youth, allure, but whose chief action would appear to be an instant depletion of our wallets.

Self-perpetuating, lubricated, chip and rot resist, permanently damp-proofed and equipped with a whole battery of built-in safety devices, to mention but a few of the virtues of normal, human skin, but what must we do to care for it? By examining its structure and functions we realise that, miraculously, the answer is very, very little!

What to choose and why

As we are beginning to realise, the cosmetic factor is, in fact, the smallest component. Yet it is a significant one for those who wish to explore the possibilities of such aid. Therapy counselling is used in conjunction with the cosmetic factor when it is felt that this will benefit the patient, or, as is so often the case, the patient's family and close relatives.

There are many cases of disfigurement. Many skin diseases even today are of unknown etiology. In this book I give guide lines from my own experience, research trials and observation over the last two decades in the muting, concealment, disguise or counter-balance of the obvious and unwanted manifestations of disease or injury, which are present as visual deviation. The sheet below is given to all patients.

THE SOCIETY OF SKIN CAMOUFLAGE AND DISFIGUREMENT THERAPY

Skin Camouflage Advice Sheet No. 1

1 *a* Always start with a clean, *dry* skin.

  b Have all items assembled before you commence as a speedy unbroken application will produce a better result.

2   Camouflage procedures vary according to the type of preparation selected, e.g. paste, liquid, cream, etc. and also in relation to the purpose of application which can be to mute, conceal or camouflage. Selected procedures are itemised separately but certain measures common to all are as follows: —

  a All powders must be allowed to set on the skin for a period of no less than ten minutes.

  b All powders, after the setting period, must be removed with a brush. This should be a long handled (for better balance and control) professional large mop (or similar from art stores).

  c Any *liquefying* cleansing cream or oil, followed by soap, preferably unperfumed (unless soap is, for any reason, contra-indicated), and water, is the most satisfactory method of removing.

3   The order in which preparations are applied is important, and your own application procedures will be detailed separately to help you. We have a common problem and are trying to share our experience and knowledge to help each other and to help the many other people with similar problems. If you are in doubt about anything or need further advice, please do not hesitate to write to

me again. Also, if you have any ideas or suggestions
on any aspect of camouflage care please contact
me so that we can share these and in doing so
provide a more helpful service for everyone.

Overall assessment

At the outset we must establish the criteria which help
to decide whether the use of cosmetic aids is likely to
be of benefit, but we must also bear in mind that there
can be no hard and fast rule in these matters for each
person is unique. For example, classification three and
four is based upon the assumption that significant outside
family relationships will, in the bulk of persons, develop
within this age group but, as in all averages, some will
be earlier and some later than in this age group.

Major age groups
1 Under fives, either sex
2 Five to eleven, either sex
3 Eleven to fifteen, boys
4 Eleven to fifteen, girls
5 Fifteen to twenty two, both sexes
6 Twenty two to thirty-five, both sexes
7 Fifty to sixty five, female
8 Fifty to sixty five, male
9 Sixty five and over, both sexes

Categories one, two, three, four and nine will often require
the active participation of other members of the family.
There will however, be an important distinction in the
case of one and two in that the non-disfigured family's
reactions may well be the sole motivation for the introduction of the cosmetic factor and the disfigured child
may have no wish for such procedures and may, even,
and quite often, actively reject and resist the use of cosmetics. The attitudes fostered in these earliest years are
vital for the child's future development and irreparable

harm can be done by the wrong approach to parent or child. The personal competence factor is a prime concern in groups one, two and nine and in all three cases perfection of result will not be the aim but a minimum cover as an aid as, and if, required.

There are many variations and causes of skin diseases/ problems and it is, therefore, highly dangerous for any person to attempt cosmetic cover or counselling, on themselves or on others, except with prior medical/psychiatric approval, referral and supervision. Accordingly, the other two categorisations that constitute the overall assessment are omitted except as references.

Nature and prognosis of condition causing disfigurement
a Burns and grafts, in many cases combined.
b Abnormal hair growth or loss.
c Skin discoloration with no alteration to contour or texture.
d Skin discoloration with disturbance of contour.
e Skin discoloration and deterioration.
f Scarring: raised or 'indented'.

Psychiatric/Psycho-somatic
a Disfigurement-crutch syndrome.
b Exaggerated concern over minimal or imagined defects.

Dear Mr Brown,

SKIN CAMOUFLAGE AND DISFIGUREMENT THERAPY CLINIC

Thank you for your enquiry. The correct procedure for you to obtain help is to ask your doctor to refer you to the Consultant Plastic Surgeon or Consultant Dermatologist at one of the hospital centres at which I hold National Health Service Clinics. The Consultant will then consider your eligibility for referral to the Camouflage Clinic. I do not have a private practice and can see people only by referral which, in the first instance, must be through your own doctor. I shall

be pleased to answer any further queries in this connection but would ask you to enclose a stamped
addressed envelope with your enquiry.

It is very helpful if patients who receive appointments
will bring with them all preparations in use at the
present time and also list carefully (brand names,
shades, types, etc.) items that have been tried in the
past together with their comments on these. If make-up
is worn *at any time,* it is important to *wear* this when
you come to see me. It is also a great help if parents
of younger children (particularly my under-five patients)
will bring with them a favourite toy or book.

With the best will in the world, it is essential for
me to meet you to be able to advise you properly for
disfigurement therapy, although it includes the cosmetic
component, it is a *total* approach to the social,
economic, family and community problems in the context of your own personality and way of life. Also, if
camouflage materials can be of help, it is important to
select, most carefully, the type of preparation suited to
your own age, skin texture and colour and to instruct
you in the easy, but specialised, application techniques,
and, if ordinary cosmetics are used, to show you how
these can be blended with camouflaging preparations.
There are no fees and no purchases involved at any
stage of this service.

You might like to know that I see my patients in
private and by appointment — you need not be shy or
feel embarrassed in any way — and that the minimum
time of your first consultation with me will be one
hour.

I will do my best to help you and look forward to
meeting you.

                      Yours sincerely,

                              DOREEN TRUST.

The next point, often overlooked, but extremely important,
is the durability factor. People who wear wigs would not
find it desirable for these to come off at lunch time, nor
when they ran for a bus. In the same way, a disfigured
person must be able to feel safe in the knowledge that
their camouflage is intact. Unless this can be assured the
wearing of cosmetics will give rise to an insecurity that,

ultimately, will be more damaging in its effect (in part, because such responses are not fully understood by the person, or his/her family) than would the more painful but straightforward adjustment to an undisguised visual deviation.

Similarly, with another group of problems, where the scarring or pitting is extremely deep. There are various complicated, lengthy, and not always very comfortable ways of concealing such problems by the use of waxes, resins etc. These, however, in practice, can create other new problems and, often, are only totally successful when carried out by a third party. This is not sensible, nor feasible, and the most helpful thing to do in such cases is to say so; effect whatever improvements can be attained, along the lines of the ideas described in an earlier chapter and attempt to inculcate coping mechanisms and a positive attitude to the problems.

Such a course of action is easier to propose than to carry out. Perhaps as a *continuing* inspiration in such cases, it is a help to remind ourselves of the gallant airmen who fought in the Battle of Britain in World War II and who, at East Grinstead Hospital, in the care of Sir Archibald McIndoe and his colleagues, achieved an even greater glory in their victory over dreadful injuries and together formed the famous Guinea Pig Club.

It is possible to do more harm than good by selecting the wrong type of cosmetic. For example, in persons prone to any allergy, it is very easy to provoke further hyper-sensitivity with haphazard self-treatment.

It cannot be over emphasised that, for any skin condition outside the 'norm' or 'dry' 'oily' 'combination' 'normal', the first and only request for help should be to your doctor/dermatologist and not to the beauty counter for random experimentation in the treatment of skin disorders is likely to be costly in more ways than one and is to be sternly resisted.

The following should assist in selection of the appropriate

preparation and so enable the maximum benefit to be derived from whatever you put on your skin.

Paints.
Many of these are aniline dyes in solution in water or alcohol. They are used to combat bacterial or fungal infection, e.g. Gentian Violet solution for infections with *candida albicans* (yeast-like organisms).

Watery lotions/water solutions.
Used to cool diffusely inflamed, broken skin surfaces. Act by evaporation and should be used frequently. e.g. Lead lotion B.P.C.

Shake lotions, watery suspensions.
Essentially, a way of applying an inert powder to the skin with additional cooling benefits as water evaporates. Dabbed on and re-applied as often as required but must not be used on wet surfaces. e.g. Calamine Lotion B.P.

Oily lotions/liniments/oily suspensions.
Contain medicaments suspended in a mixture of oil and water. Many kinds. Used a great deal in dermatological practice. e.g. Calamine lotion oily B.P.C. (calamine powder, arachis oil and lime water).

Ointments
Essentially greasy preparations as they are mixtures of greases and fats. They adhere well and give protection but prevent both heat loss and evaporation and are difficult to remove except with oil or detergent, especially on hairy surfaces, and so their use is restricted to specific purposes (e.g. to soften 'crusts') and as vehicles (e.g. Emulsifying B.P.)

Ointments can be sub-divided into three types:
a Those which are completely water soluble and provide

non-staining bases of varying consistency, e.g. Nystatin ointment B.P.

b Emulsifying ointments which are used to effect intimate contact of various substances with the skin and contain either mineral oil, and an emulsifying wax, or an animal fat such as lanolin. e.g. Wool alcohols ointment.

c Non-emulsifying ointments which are occlusive and macerate the skin surface and are used only to treat chronic dry skin lesions. e.g. Paraffin ointment, Simple ointment.

Creams

Creams can be used to cool, moisten, cleanse, soften and protect the skin and are varying proportions of oil and water, emulsified, so that the ingredients do not separate out. The proportions determine the greasiness or otherwise of the end product. A dry skin is short of water, not of oil and oily substances are used to provide a protective seal to reduce evaporation of water, i.e. keep the skin's own natural moisture in. Creams are emulsions either of water dispersed in oil (water-in-oil) or of oil dispersed in water (oil-in-water).

Oil-in-water creams

These creams are especially useful as vehicles for water soluble substances (e.g. Buffered cream B.N.F.) and are the cosmetic type vanishing creams.

Water-in-oil creams

These are not easily washed off and behave and feel like oils but are more cosmetically acceptable than ointments as the water content makes them spread more readily. Such creams are useful for protecting the skin when it is chapped and dried or on a baby's buttocks. They can be used on hairy skin surfaces without dragging and can be used as vehicles, for fat soluble substances particularly. e.g. Oily cream B.P. which is water-in-oil emulsion containing water and Wool alcohols ointment.

Barrier creams

The composition of proprietary barrier creams is complex, but silicones and soaps and talc seem to be important ingredients. Barrier creams may make it easier to clean the skin after dirty work but they should be readily removable, otherwise skin irritations and hypersensitivity reactions may occur due to blocked sweat glands and follicles.

Masking creams

These are for the temporary obscuring of skin blemishes. Again, there are various kinds, some of which may consist of inert Titanium Oxide, ointment base and suitable colourings. They should always be thoroughly removed from skin.

Powders

They reduce unnecessary skin friction, alleviate itching; are used to apply anti-bacterial and anti-fungal agents to the skin, cool by increasing effective surface area; cosmetically, to impart bloom, reduce or increase shine, highlight, shade, enhance and 'fix' and thicken various preparations. Water repellent powders such as zinc stearate powder B.N.F. can be used on babies. Basic ingredients used separately or in many combinations. e.g. talc, most lubricant and does not absorb water. Starch, less lubricant and absorbs water.

SPECIAL INFORMATION TABLE

Brushes

1 Think of the brushes you use as the physical extension of your fingers.
2 Care for them properly, like this:
   a Wet brush in warm water.
   b Rub lightly on a cake of white laundry soap.
   c Rub bristles on palm of hand until lather is made and all colour is completely out.
   d Rinse thoroughly in warm water.
   e Squeeze damp brush lightly between thumb and fingers to shape up bristles so that they dry into the correct form.

Pastes

Preparations containing insoluble powders in an ointment base, the term being usually restricted to preparations in which the amount of powder is of the order of 25% or more. Pastes usually contain zinc oxide, starch, soft paraffin and other active substances can be incorporated. Pastes are protective, adhesive and emollient. e.g. Zinc gelatin B.P. (Unna's paste).

SPECIAL INFORMATION TABLE

Underpainting

a Either to show through a subsequent layer of paint,
   or
b to alter the colours applied over it.

For example, a bright yellow underpaint with, say, a thin layer of blue will produce a green of greater luminosity and provide a more effective and natural camouflage than one thick layer of a green colour.

Know your oils

Olive oil

A pale yellow or greenish-yellow oil expressed from ripe olives. There are several grades available, the best and first pressing is termed 'virgin oil'. Dermatologically innocuous and a very useful emollient. It is widely used in cosmetics of all kinds.

Avocado pear oil, Alligator pear oil

A green oil obtained from the fleshy portions of the avocado pear. It is emollient and dermatologically innocuous; used in cosmetic oils and lubricating creams because, it is claimed, it possesses special characteristics. According to R. G. Harry in *Cosmetic Materials,* 'extensive investigation and controlled dermatological tests are necessary to establish whether or not this oil has any

F

beneficial properties other than those exerted by any other emollient oil on the skin.

Turtle oil
Turtle oil is often obtained from the muscles and genital organs of the giant sea turtle, reputedly from two hundred and fifty to seven hundred years old, and is found in Mexican waters. It is used in lubricating wrinkle creams etc. In extensive investigations reported in *British Journal Dermatology,* no evidence was found to suggest that turtle oil possessed dermatological qualities superior to the useful, innocuous and emollient properties of other fish, e.g. cod liver oil and vegetable oils.

Palm oil
Obtained from the ripe fruit of the palm tree. Bleached palm oil is dermatologically innocuous and is used in the manufacture of mild toilet soaps and household soaps.

Arachis oil, Peanut oil, Groundnut oil
Expressed from the seeds. It is often used as a substitute for olive or almond oils in cosmetic creams, anti-wrinkle oils etc. A useful emollient, which is dermatologically innocuous.

Mineral oils, Petroleum oils, including Liquid paraffin
Clear, oily liquids obtained from petroleum oil from which the waxes (petroleum jelly, paraffin wax) have been removed and the more volatile fractions (benzine, kerosene etc.) have been distilled. These are inexpensive and therefore are widely used in extensive ranges of cosmetics. Properly prepared mineral oils are dermatologically innocuous, lacking in skin penetration in the absence of wetting agents. They are also useful surface emollients.

Experiments on skin penetration, *(British Journal Dermatology)* found no evidence of any appreciable difference between the absorption of different vegetable oils, Arachis, Avocado, Castor, Grapeseed, Olive and of Turtle oil. This group of oils had less penetrant properties than Cod liver oil, Lanolin etc. and both these groups had penetrant properties not possessed by the mineral oils.

Some basic setting powders. Average, 1976 price of each is in the region of 25p per 100g.

Formula 'A'

Light Magnesium Carbonate	5g
Magnesium Stearate	5g
Titanium Dioxide	5g
Strontium Carbonate	10g
Zinc Oxide	10g
French Chalk to:	100g

Formula 'B'

Light Magnesium Carbonate	5g
Magnesium Stearate	5g
Zinc Stearate	5g
Light Kaolin	5g
Zinc Oxide	5g
Titanium Dioxide	5g
Strontium Carbonate	10g
French Chalk to:	100g

Formula 'C'

Light Magnesium Carbonate	5g
Magnesium Stearate	5g
Calcium Carbonate	5g
Strontium Carbonate	5g
Zinc Oxide	5g
Titanium Dioxide	10g
French Chalk to:	100g

Prosthetic aids

The 'face-maker's clay', is how one surgeon refers to the acrilyc compounds from which many prostheses are created today, and prosthetic devices of many kinds can replace missing parts of the body, such as the breast, upper and lower limbs, nose, eyes and various dental prostheses.

Hunting and tribal war wounds, punitive mutilations and disease were a physical and social handicap for early man, just as they are for us today and records indicate that they used a variety of ingenious and exotic materials to attempt reconstruction of the physiognomy. Nasal pros-

theses were made of lacquer in India and China in the
second century and artificial eyes, noses and ears have
been found in the graves of Egyptian mummies. It was,
however, not until the fifteenth century and the advent
of surgeons Ambroise Paré and Gasparo Togliocozzi that
the continuing development of these methods was clearly
recorded. In 1579 Paré described his approach to prosthetic
reconstruction of the nose:

> *'By what means a part of the nose is cut off may be
> restored, or how instead of the nose that is cut off
> another counterfeit nose may be fastened or placed in
> the stead'*
>
> 'When the whole nose is cut off from the face or
> portion of the nostrils from the nose, it cannot be
> restored or joined again for it is not in men as in
> plants. Instead of the nose cut away or consumed, it
> is requisite to substitute another made by art because
> that nature cannot supply that defect, this nose so
> artificially made must be of gold, silver, paper or linen
> cloths glued together; it must be so coloured, counter-
> feited and made both of fashion, figure and bigness,
> that it may as aptly as is possible resemble the natural
> nose; it must be bound or staid on with little threads
> or laces unto the hinder part of the head or the hat.
> Also if there be any portion of the upper lip cut off
> with the nose, you may shadow it with annexing some
> such things that is wanting unto the nose, and cover
> it with hair on his upper lip that he may not want
> anything that may adorn or beautify the face'.

Many of his prostheses were of a marvellous ingenuity,
eyes made of gold and silver 'counterfeited and enamelled
to have brightness and gemmy decency of the natural eye'
and were often held in place by bands of gold and silver
wire encircling the head.

In the course of this century many materials have been
used for facial prostheses — including vulcanite, celluloid,
aluminium, silver, gelatin glycerine compounds, pre-
vulcanised latex, silicone rubbers of many kinds and
plastics such as poly-methyl methacrylate, and experi-

mentation continues. It is not possible within the confines of this book to elaborate further or to discuss experimentations over many years but there is a wealth of technical data available in many excellent books. The American Academy of Maxillo-facial Prosthetics was formed in 1951 'for the purpose of pooling the technical knowledge and experience of its members and to provide a centre of information that may be needed by other workers interested in this field'.

The period from the two World Wars has seen a resurgence of interest in the prosthetic restoration of maxillo facial deformities and the use of new materials and refined techniques has added impetus, but despite such advances, one of the leading workers in this field. in a superb, recently published book says:

> Unfortunately, some people consider it a stigma to wear anything that is false, particularly if the object is exposed to view. This unjustifiable and often very unfair deterrent to the confident use of a prosthesis can and should be overcome. A facial prosthesis not only must be usable, but must pass unnoticed and be in total harmony with the patient's features and acceptable to the general public.

That our society *is* capable of changing its attitudes to external aids is shown in the fact that the wearing of dentures and spectacles is seen today as a normal, socially acceptable necessity to which no stigma attaches and bespectacled 'beauties' such as Bardot, Loren and Princess Grace of Monaco prove just how far we have come and just how fast public attitudes *can* be changed from the days of Dorothy Parker and 'Men never make passes at girls who wear glasses'.

As Doctor Bulbulian says in his book, 'likewise, any other type of intraoral or extraoral restoration that benefits the patient physically, psychologically and economically should be accepted in the same manner, but unfortunately it is not always so accepted'.

It is interesting to note that artificial aids, when fashionably, intentionally promoted, can find public acceptance, even when these are abused and frivolously exploited as is shown in the admiring acceptance of a variety of 'paddings' to attain a 'desirable' outline, or the open flaunting of plastic propped pneumatics in the pages of *Playboy* and others of that ilk. In the light of this, it is a sad reflection on us as a society that we do not expend a similar amount of energy on the promotion of a public appearance and tolerance in areas where man-made devices are a bridge to *normality* itself, rather than an optional extra.

In 1974 it was estimated that there were more than 100,000 permanent colostomies in Great Britain, with one colostomy for every 4,000 members of the population of which two thirds would be permanent, and yet Consultant Surgeon, Mr H. B. Devlin, in a lecture given at the 59th London Nursing Exhibition that same year, pointed out that fifty per cent of patients with colostomies (as opposed to ten per cent in a study of 'normal' elderly patients) became socially isolated: —

> 'Yet another indication that the colostomy patients are stigmatised by society or more probably stigmatised by themselves. Colostomy patients have many problems to contend with. They have the problem of the operation, they have psychological and social problems and many of them feel stigmatised and different from the rest of society. Much can be done to help them but helping them implies setting up a service to look after them and *identify their problems*. This nowadays means finding resources and using them expeditiously'.

The colostomy patient can camouflage his condition by wearing clothes and so appearing whole and normal to his family and the outside world. His battle is fought in private.

The facial mutilee is forced to exhibit his condition. His

own public face is his own public battleground. The facial mutilee has no privacy and no escape.

Surgeons can perform miracles of healing and reconstruction. Under certain circumstances, however, surgery and/or further surgery is not feasible nor likely to produce a more acceptable result and when this occurs, a prosthetic procedure can be recommended, often with gratifyingly beneficial results for the patient. The continuing development of new materials indicates that the scope of and demand for prostheses will increase and as attention focuses on the question of face and identity, sympathetic and perceptive surgeons increasingly prescribe facial prostheses. Roberts (1971) says 'The construction of a facial restoration requires technical skill and artistic abilities. The qualities involved are those of artist, chemist and engineer. To combine these specialities requires a person who is trained to use a wide range of materials and apply them to the problem of facial restoration'.

Although technical and functional efficiency are prime requisites, the success or failure of a facial restoration can only rest solely on whether or not it fulfils its main purpose *as desired by the patient.*

Many film and stage processes and materials can produce splendid prosthetic results and can be a useful source of inspiration but it should always be remembered that these are created for temporary application to a whole structure and healthy skin. The continuously worn medical prosthesis requires that aesthetic finesse should be based on and tempered by an awareness of underlying problems and the use of only rigorously screened, safe and medically approved materials.

Natural appearance, reasonable durability and comfort in wear are essential for a successful prosthesis; the other cardinal requirements are ease of application and comfortable retention and skin adhesives are one aspect of this.

The qualities required in a skin adhesive are that it should be:

non-irritant
non-toxic
easy to apply
easy to remove without injuring the skin
compatible with type of material used for prosthesis
unlikely to affect appearance or durability or prosthesis
retentive for day-long wear
portable in small quantity for emergency use

There are various types of skin adhesive:

Liquid
Silicone Spray-on
Latex paste type
Double-coated adhesive tapes

Liquid Adhesives
These are commonly known as spirit-gum adhesives and used for many years in the theatre. The basic ingredients of this are mastic gum dissolved in a solvent such as ether and/or some form of alcohol. An effective and inexpensive spirit gum formulation can be:

Compound Mastic paint BPC
Mastic 40%
Castor Oil 1.25%
Benzole Nitration grade of commerce to 100%

This can be removed with exylene or ether. Matt adhesive is a proprietary non-shining type of spirit gum.

Double-sided adhesive tapes
This is attached and cut to fit the prosthesis first and then positioned on the face. Easy to handle but may have to be changed quite frequently as it obviously loses some of its adhesive power after each application. There are various brands; some seem more flexible and easier to apply. Cleanly removed by peeling from prosthesis or skin.

Silicone spray-on
Polysilixane pressure-sensitive polymer in a fluorocarbon
propellant. It is applied by spraying-on. A special remover
is required. There are many types available.

Latex paste type
Formulated from natural rubber, zinc oxide and solvents.
Tubes of paste give ease of application. The 'surgical
cement' used for fixing appliances such as ilcostomy and
colostomy bags. They can be removed with xylene or
ether. Many brands are available. Certain types of latex
eyelash adhesive in sealed, small and easily portable tubes
can be useful in case of emergency. To give a better finish
to the edge, stipple with a sponge-tip applicator.

The use of adhesive is contra-indicated in some cases
and the material from which the prosthesis is constructed
together with its type and location may restrict the
possible choice of adhesive. When the use of an adhesive
has been approved it is advisable to experiment with the
range of permitted preparations to find the most satisfactory in every way, which must always include the application and removal of the prosthesis *without* professional
assistance.

In this, as in all 'camouflage' techniques, no help is better
than bad help. Bulbulian (1945) says in this respect:

> 'In case of failure, after many hours of labour, it still
> is far better to be frank with the patient, to tell him of
> the failure and not to subject him to the possible
> humiliation of wearing an unsatisfactory prosthesis
> (face) in public. *A prosthesis that merely converts a
> pathetic condition to a comical one is worse than no
> prosthesis at all.* A person who has gone through such
> a discouraging experience may become so sensitive to
> the idea of wearing a prosthesis that he subsequently
> may be reluctant to accept and wear even a well-made
> restoration'.

6: QUESTIONS AND ANSWERS

Some of your questions answered

*Every morning I see a part of me that the world has no idea of
and I feel horrified and ashamed.*

Q. I have *acne-like* spots that will not go although I have spent a fortune on different creams and 'cures'. Could you please tell me what to use?

A. No. Nor should you experiment further. In your own interest, do not seek nor accept, the advice of anyone else except your own Doctor and/or Skin Specialist (and by that I mean a medically qualified Dermatologist). Acne vulgaris can be simulated by papulo-pustular reactions to some drugs, such as oral contraceptives, androgens, halogens and corticosteroids, whether these are prescribed for oral or local use. The absence of comedones (blackheads), unusual distribution and the patient's age are differentiating factors and your own Doctor the person best fitted to advise you. Let me know of your progress.

Q. What do you feel about giving the 'Pill' to a twelve-year-old to prevent acne?

A. There are many useful standard precautions to try for the treatment of acne before resorting to more complicated medication and it is rare for a twelve-year-old to suffer acne as the hormone levels are not yet established. Some dermatologists have used oestrogens in the treatment of acne vulgaris and contraceptive pills are generally well tolerated but their use by adolescents might be thought to raise issues beyond medical treatment alone. I do not believe in random, haphazard self-medication and would urge that you consult your own doctor and take his advice on any such matter.

Q. I have been using *aerosols* for some time now and although they are easier it is very annoying as so often there seems to be a lot left in the can that will not come out. Why does this happen and can I puncture the tin to get the rest out?

A. Despite modern controls and testing some faulty aerosols seem to get through, and the manufacturers will usually replace the faulty item if you return it to them. An aerosol is designed to expel its total contents and it is usually mis-use that prevents it from doing so. Many aerosol products are designed to be shaken before you use them as the formulation used may separate into its constituents and failure to do this dispenses an unsatisfactory product and also means there will probably be a residue left in the can. Using the aerosol in an inverted or horizontal position, unless the instructions indicate this, will also mean there will be some left as many aerosols contain a dip tube which reaches to the bottom of the can and when the can is inverted propellant gas will be dispensed and will therefore be unable to dispense all the product. Abnormally low temperatures can impair an aerosol's efficiency, although some are specially made to function at low temperature, and they should of course, be stored away from sources of heat. This includes being left in sunlight or on radiator shelves, as this causes their contents to expand and increases their internal pressure and, if excessive, can cause them to burst. No, you should not attempt to puncture any aerosol as this is both a very messy and hazardous procedure which should never be done except under controlled laboratory conditions.

Q. I have been told that I should not use things containing lanolin but I just do not understand why as I have been using lanolin cream for years now until I had this skin trouble. Does it mean that I never have to use lanolin again or just stop using it for a time? As it does not say on the jars and tubes, how do I know whether things have lanolin in them or not?

A. In view of the wide-spread use of potential sensitising agents, the skin performs its protective function rather well. However, it is a fact that one can *develop* a sensitivity to anything at any time, though the reasons for this are not always known.

Once an allergy is established it means that contact with the offending substance must at all times be avoided and, yes, this means always, not just temporarily. Recent work indicates that lanolin sensitivity is on the increase.

Lanolin is used in many cosmetics and even skin medicaments. It appears under a number of names: e.g. Wool Fat; Cera Lanae, Adeps Lanae; as you probably know already, it is obtained from the wool of sheep. As your own request for lanolin-free preparations has been echoed by a number of readers I am compiling an up-to-date list and hope to publish this in *Talkabout* quite soon.

Allergies are myth, mystery and to those who suffer them, painful realities and there are now special clinics and highly specialised and sophisticated testing techniques. Even so, the possibility that some skin problems can be allergic in origin is sometimes overlooked as one Dermatologist remarks, 'It takes a knowing eye, a suspicious mind and very often long questioning and testing to prove it'. An easy-to-follow book on this subject is *'Hypersensitivity: Mechanisms and Management'*, William B. Sherman (1968). *The Practitioner* review of January 1969 referred to the book as 'a book of distinction . . . strongly recommended'.

Q. How many different types of birthmark are there?
A. At least ten. Terminology is a little confusing for the lay person. *Naevus* is often used to denote birthmarks of all types. Vascular birthmarks (Haemangiomata) are very common and divide into different types:
Capillary haemangioma (Port wine stain; Naevus

flammeus; Flat haemangioma): This is a circumscribed defect of dermal capillaries which are dilated; present in its full extent at birth; usually unilateral on face or neck but other, and very large areas may be affected; does not disappear spontaneously; as yet, no totally satisfactory curative treatment; covering creams usually extremely effective on this type of blemish.

Cavernous haemangioma (Strawberry mark): Simple haemangioma: An increase and dilation of capillaries: bright red, raised, sharply circumscribed, can be partly blanched by compression; absent or present only as a minute red dot at birth it appears within the first few weeks of life and grows rapidly for the first few months; varied in size up to medium-large strawberry and is usually single; can occur anywhere but most often on head and neck; usually left untreated as the great majority of cases involute spontaneously over a period of several years; minor plastic surgery to remove skin-folds is occasionally required when spontaneous resolution has been completed. I do not recommend the use of covering creams initially, but these can be used on reaching a certain stage of involution and this is, usually, before the child starts school. Some cavernous haemangioma are entirely subcutaneous and present as an irregular, bluish-red, compressible swelling over parts of which the skin itself may be normal: occasionally superficial (simple type) and deep components are present in the same lesion.

Spider naevus: A central bright red spot from which thread-like dilated blood vessels radiate; the whole about 1 cm in diameter. Not commonly seen on the face in childhood and adolescence; often appear for the first time in pregnancy, and disappear again afterwards; without significance and do not require treatment except for cosmetic reasons when they can be removed by destruction of the central vessel by diathermy or cautery; easily concealed with camouflage preparations.

Naevi in one form or another are extremely common and are found in 95 per cent of adults. Quite the most interesting book I read on this subject is *Vascular Spiders and Related Lesions of the Skin* by William Bennett Bean (1959). This was most favourably reviewed in the *British Journal of Dermatology*, October, 1960.

Q. For about five months now I have had funny brownish-patches on my face and the skin is roughish. I have been to all sorts of beauty counters and people for advice and have jars and jars of all sorts of creams for dry skin but they do not seem to do me any good at all. I would feel so silly trying to tell my Doctor as it does not seem very serious but really I am worried sick in case I have some awful complaint.

A. I suggest, first, that you resolve to stop buying expensive cosmetics for none of these will make one iota of difference to anything, except your bank account. Secondly, if you really and truly are unable to discuss your problem with your doctor ask him to refer you for a private consultation with a Dermatologist. I really do understand just how you feel, but remember that, with all his skill and knowledge, the Doctor and/or Dermatologist can only help your problem and understand your feelings if you explain them first. The *bran-like eruptions* are symptomatic of a commonly occurring problem so you have no need to be frightened, but you do need to get proper medical diagnosis and treatment.

Q. I recently entered into correspondence with the advertisers of a *breast-developing cream* who informed me that it contained 'a hormone' and that this was within 'the safety limits set down by the Department of Trade and Industry'. Could you tell me what this means?

A. Oestrogenic substances in the form of external preparations such as this and other similar creams should only be sold from a Pharmacy as they are classed as Part I poisons. However, if a cream contains *less* than four milligrams of oestrogen per 100g of cream, it is considered a safe limit by the Poisons Board which administers these controls as it may then be sold by anyone, which includes mail-order companies. My personal advice:

a never undertake anything of this nature without first consulting your own doctor and

b as you are so unhappy and determined to do something, why not try something such as breathing and posture-improvements that will help to improve your *whole* figure as well as your bustline?

Q. Could you tell me what something called a *catatonic* detergent is and does?

A. There is more than one. The catatonic detergents or quaternary ammonium compounds, are compatible with each other but incompatible with soap. They are bactericidal and have the property of lowering surface tension which allows grease to be removed and so they are used for cleansing infected areas. For example, you will probably have heard of Savlon which is a proprietary preparation of the catatonic detergent Centrimide BP/CTAB, Cetavlon — 3 per cent and chlorhexidine 0.3 per cent.

Q. Can I wear my own ordinary cosmetics if I wear a covering cream?

A. Your own favourite type of cosmetic can be applied, in the usual way into and/or over camouflage preparations.

G

Q. What does your service *cost?*

A. The NHS Skin Camouflage Service is freely available to all who are in need of care.

Q. Are *covering creams* waterproof?

A. Some of the covering creams are waterproof providing that the application instructions are properly observed.

Q. I feel so *depressed* about the way I look and I started having a drink just to cheer myself up. Somehow I cannot seem to stop now and yet I am so ashamed of myself I cannot bring myself to tell my husband and I dare not go to the doctor just because I am too weak-willed. I do not know who to turn to and cannot seem to pull myself together.

A. Do not under-estimate yourself. You have already taken the first step in pulling yourself together by writing to me . . . a positive step. It seems, from the long list of preparations, that you are using far too many things and I have sent you a simplified routine and detailed the order and manner in which you should use everything. You will save time and get a better result. I cannot advise you more until I see you in person and you will find the appointment procedure outlined in the newsletter. Incidentally, you will find that there is a much greater understanding of the problem of alcoholism than perhaps you realise. Indeed, the organisation *Alcoholics Anonymous* is made up of people who themselves have been alcoholic at some time in their lives and so have a *real,* first hand understanding of the problems and offer help, support and guidance.

Q. My lips are very *dry* and cracked and sometimes they get very sore and seem to peel. Can you suggest anything to help?

A. You do not tell me whether this is a current or permanent problem. Dry, cracked lips can be a seasonable hazard and the use of a lip-salve should speedily resolve this type of problem. Lip-salves are inexpensive (from 7p upwards) and are available in colourless or, slightly tinted, lipstick form. There is also a colourless cream called Blisteze which can be worn under your normal lipstick. It is also possible that you are licking your lips and causing your own problem. Many people have this habit. Wearing a tinted or colourless high gloss over your usual lipstick would, by texture sensation, make you aware of the action and enable you to break the habit. It is also possible that your problem could be caused by a reaction against substances in your lipstick. Some ordinary lipsticks can be obtained in an unperfumed version if perfume is the irritant. A major chemist chain-store produce a 'Special Formula' lipstick. There is also a special Lip Barrier Cream to wear under lipstick. Finally, there is a special sun-screen lip preparation. If the problem is merely a seasonal one, the regular use of a lip-salve and/or gloss should improve the condition within a few days. If, however, this is a persistent, constantly recurring problem you should seek the advice of your own doctor.

Q. My young son has protruding *ears* and has always been very self-conscious about them. He has become so depressed about this lately that he refuses to go out with his friends any more. He will not go, with or without me, to see the doctor in case he thinks he is cissy. I have talked about the problem with friends but I seem to get so many different suggestions that I just do not know what to do for the best any more. I have heard that there is an operation for protruding ears nowadays and wonder if you can tell me anything about this. How long do you have to wear bandages and stay in hospital? I worry so much

about this for him and I often feel guilty in case
it is all my fault for letting him lie on his side when
he was young.

A. I understand. Be at peace in your mind and rest
assured that you are in no way responsible. The cause
is congenital and is the over-development of cartilage
in the region of the ear called the concha. The corrective operation is done through an incision behind
the ear at its junction with the skull. The excess
cartilage and skin are removed so that the ear aligns
correctly and the incision repaired with very fine
stitches. A Plastic Surgeon comments as follows on
the other points:

> 'The outer surface of the ear may appear swollen and
> bruised for two to three weeks. Dressings are removed
> two to three days after the operation although it is
> advisable, particularly in the case of a young, or rest-
> less sleeper, to wear a bandage round the ears in bed
> for some time afterwards. The stitches behind the ears
> are removed in seven to eight days and the hair may
> be washed one week after the stitches have been
> removed. The period of hospitalisation is the decision
> of the surgeon but the minimum period would be two
> days'.

My own feeling on this is that you should go, on your
own, to have a quiet chat with your family doctor. I
realise from the remainder of your letter that you
are afraid of being brusquely dismissed and made to
feel foolish but I would ask you not to let this fear
deter you from seeking help. I think you will find
that your own doctor will be sympathetic and do all
that he can to help you and your son.

Q. My eyelashes are now so very light that I just have
to wear mascara. I use a brown mascara and *eye liner*
but always seem to be left with a space between the
liner and mascara and when I try to fill it in the

mascara gets into my eyes which makes me blink a lot and then all my make-up smudges. I cannot think what I do wrong as I have tried so often to get it right.

A. First of all, you do not have to wear mascara, you could use an eyelash tint or switch to false eyelashes. However, just in case for any reason you cannot, or do not wish to use either of above ideas, let us return to mascara. I would hazard a guess, in view of the fact that you have tried without success so often, that you are merely sitting wrongly. A reason so simple that it is overlooked. So, position is important. Look down your nose into a mirror, so that the eyes are relaxed when you are applying your liner. You will have to practise this part, as dexterity in this is hard to acquire, but do check that you are using a sufficiently firm, fine brush and remember that one with a long handle will give you an easier control and balance. Also, a brown-black liner will give you better definition. Finally, fold a tissue in half and just place this under your lashes before you start and while you work so that, if you do blink, you will blink on this rather than your face, with the result of having no more make-up smears.

Q. My daughter, living in Sheffield, has written to tell me that her Doctor has told her to use *glass-paper pads* on her face to keep down the excessive hair growth. She says that it is making her face very sore but she will not go back to see the Doctor in case he thinks she is making a lot of fuss over such a small problem.

A. It is not quite so horrific as you fear as the glass-paper pads referred to are very fine and are, I assure you, specially made for the purpose of the removal of unwanted hair. These pads are usually employed on legs and arms and great care must be exercised when using them on the face. I suggest that your daughter temporarily discontinues the use of this on her face and, instead, practises on her forearm for at least a week until she is accustomed to handling the pad and thereby able to control the pressure she exerts when using it. Then I suggest that she graduates to a small, less obvious part of her face, eventually encompassing the whole area to be treated. The movements should be light and rapid. We should all remember never to use the face as a 'testing site' for any new product or procedure.

Q. I seem to have developed an allergy to a *hair* dye I am using. Does this mean I will not ever be able to use it again?

A. You will probably find that you are allergic to one component of your hair dye and you must never come into contact with that again. Special skin testing by a dermatologist would probably be able to identify the offending substance and then, if you wish to dye your hair you should find a preparation that does not contain the offending substances or derivatives. There are now some 6,000 ingredients used in the cosmetics industry and new ones are being added to this. It is my own belief that manufacturers of cosmetics should be compelled to disclose the content of their preparations in the same way that the manufacturers of medical preparations do. In the meantime try patch testing and use the hair dye, sparingly.

Q. I have neglected my *hands* terribly and they are so rough and wrinkled now that I am really ashamed of them. I vaguely remember reading somewhere about wax treatments and wonder if this would help me? I would have to do it myself as I have three children and cannot afford to spend very much on myself.

A. The material used for this is chemically pure paraffin, which is melted and retained at a temperature of

140° - 175°. The melted wax is sprayed or brushed onto the skin and, after being hermetically sealed, left for periods of 10-60 minutes. Its uses include all over body treatments; localised applications on hands or feet; and in various facial treatments. There is no reason why you should not do this yourself if you are quite sure that yours is merely a problem of continued neglect and I am sending you detailed instructions under separate cover. From the tone of your letter I imagine that your children are quite young and I would suggest that you do not attempt any such treatment on yourself unless you are quite sure that you have sufficient, uninterrupted time at your disposal. Meantime, you could check that you are not using too harsh a washing detergent and perhaps wear rubber/household gloves for domestic chores and also, the frequent use of a bland emollient cream would be beneficial and I would suggest E45 cream, purchased from the drug counter of most chemists.

Q. I notice that some of the things I buy at the chemists have *letters* after the name of the product and I would like to know what it means as they are sometimes different and it is confusing?

A. Yes, I agree, it does all seem a bit mysterious. Some items have B.N.F. which stands for British National Formulary and is the National Health Service prescription book issued for doctors; B.P., British Pharmacopeia and B.P.C., British Pharmaceutical Codex are also used. The purpose, and advantage, of attaching these letters is so that you will be able to obtain the same product from any chemist or pharmacy wherever you are as these letters guarantee that the item has been dispensed in accordance with a nationally recognised standard and method.

Q. Can *moles,* birthmarks and similar blemishes be treated surgically?

A. Sometimes. This depends upon the type of blemish, how big it is and where it is located. Your Doctor and Consultant Plastic Surgeon and/or Consultant Dermatologist are the correct source of advice on all such matters.

Q. I have been told that an *oatmeal bath* would do me good but it sounds such a horrid and messy idea. Is there some special way of taking an oatmeal bath?

A. There are a number of ways! In my opinion, the most pleasant and efficient is as follows.

  a Tie hair firmly out of way and/or wear a well-fitting shower cap.

  b Place a good handful of oatmeal into a 'sock' made out of tubular gauze and then tie up open end.

  c Hold (or fix firmly) underneath the hot water tap and fill bath to desired level. The oatmeal swells and the flowing water washes out a turbid solution of oatmeal starch.

  d When bath is suitably filled and at a comfortable temperature, get in and 'soap' yourself all over using oatmeal sock instead of soap.

  e Gently towel yourself dry.

This is a relaxing and comforting bath but it has an added benefit for anyone with *psoriasis* as it gently assists in the removal of excess tar and scales.

Q. I had to have an *operation* some years ago and most of the time I was scared out of my wits as I overheard myself or rather my condition discussed and just could not understand the words or what it was all supposed to mean. I am getting symptoms that bother me and feel I should go to the Doctor but I do not know how to describe what is happening and I would feel such a fool fumbling for the correct words. Is there a book I could read that is not too complicated?

A. I would advise you to look at one or two of the very reasonably priced, soft back Anatomy books written for nurses. For example, *Anatomy and Physiology for Nurses* by Evelyn Pearce, Faber. Or there is the Nurses' Aid Series *Anatomy and Physiology for Nurses* by Katherine F. Armstrong, Balliere Tindal. I think that we are often inhibited by what we feel is a lack of knowledge of the correct terminology and the reputed Chinese idea of sticking pins into a 'dummy' patient to show just where it hurts most often seems to be a good idea to many people. Perhaps it helps to remember, at such times, that before he became a Doctor, your Doctor was *also* a patient of someone, with probably just the same worries himself.

Q. When we were on holiday abroad recently the slightest bit of sunshine made my skin feel as if it were on fire. I have been having antibiotic treatment and wonder if such things can really alter the skin?

A. Yes, sometimes. It is sometimes forgotten that the skin is, in fact, the largest organ of the body, in a constant state of activity and reflecting the state of the body it covers and from which it is nourished, and this includes its medication. Iatrogenic dermatoses are quite common. Indeed, some years ago, a report from the John Hopkins Hospital pointed out that four per cent of admissions were for such reactions.

The side-effects of some antibiotics can include *photosensitivity*. Briefly, light sensitivity reactions are usually confined to the areas exposed to light and occur, in some individuals only, following both the use of certain drugs and the exposure to light of specific wavelength.

Reactions are usually classified as Phototoxic (furocoumarins and coal tar derivatives are photo-

toxic agents) or Photo-allergic (sulphonamide group,
thiazide diuretics). Photo-cross-sensitisation may sometimes occur between phenothiazine derivatives and
halogenated salicylamides and related compounds some
of which are used or have been used as antiseptics
or deodorants. You should, without further delay,
consult your own Doctor so that you can happily
and *safely* enjoy your next holiday.

Q.   I think that I have a very rare problem. I am a man
of twenty-seven and have what my doctor says are
ingrowing hairs on my face. Shaving can be quite
painful.

A.   One of the accepted treatments for *pili recurvation*
is the use of a depilatory lotion, but you must pre-
test and follow the instructions with care and precision.
A permanent and therefore perhaps preferable solution
would be to have the hair removed by electrolysis.
Men quite often and for a variety of reasons, have
the whole of their beard area made completely and
permanently hair-free. It is a slow and costly procedure but might seem worth it for a life without
shaving.

Q.   Is this sort of preparation difficult to *remove?*

A.   Covering preparations are easily removed if the correct
type of cleanser is used: Any liquefying cleansing
cream; most oils and, unless soap is contra-indicated
for any reason, soap and water to follow either cream
or oil will satisfactorily remove all covering creams.

Q.   I have half a bottle of lotion left from some I was
given to use about two years ago. Is it still *safe* to
use?

A.   You do not tell me what the lotion is or in what conditions you have been keeping it . . . light and
temperature changes can accelerate the deterioration

processes and affect potency. I would advise you to check with your Doctor before recommencing use of the preparation after so long a time. It is even possible that there will be something available that will be an improvement on the original prescription. Drugs deteriorate when stored and it might be useful to bear the following in mind for future reference:

Avoid the use of:

Any substance, liquid or solid, which has changed colour.

A clear liquid which has become cloudy or now has a sediment.

Any preparations that have passed a given expiry date.

Anything which is inadequately labelled as drugs can come in varying strengths and the dosage/application frequency will vary accordingly.

Anything that raises the slightest doubt in your mind . . . after all, you can always write to *Talkabout* now . . .

For instance, several diseases may be treated with the same drug but the dosage and way in which the drug is administered may be varied and will be carefully controlled for each condition, e.g. Stilboestrol dosage can vary from as low as 1 mg to suppress lacation to 5 mg for acne and 25 mg in carcinoma of the prostrate.

Q. My skin is in a dreadful state. I went to see a beautician and was told that I had acne and that a *skin-peeling* would help me. It is very expensive and would cost about £200. I cannot really afford it all but I am so unhappy that I am thinking of trying to borrow the money. I just feel that I would do anything to get my face looking right again. Do you think I should have it done?

A. It is extremely inadvisable to expose yourself to the
      hazards of such a treatment unless it is administered
      by someone holding the Surgical or Dermatological
      Consultant status of this country. I will quote a well
      known Consultant Dermatologist on just this pro-
      cedure: 'Lay operators have brought *secret* formulae
      over from Europe and used them to perform peeling
      procedures without having adequate knowledge of
      the penetrability, toxicity or potency of their agents'.
      We can perhaps appreciate the dangers of 'lay' treat-
      ments in this field when we know that these secret
      formulae contain agents such as liquid phenol,
      resorcinal, salicylic acid. It is true, incredibly, that
      commercial beauty clinics are allowed to advertise,
      sell and even act as agents for foreign operators who
      perform this treatment. In my opinion, it is highly
      irresponsible for anyone without the proper medical
      qualifications referred to above, to dabble in such
      matters and to do so can only indicate gross cupidity
      and a total lack of concern for the safety of the
      patient and professional ethics. Chemical Skin-Peeling
      and Dermabrasion, when considered likely to be of
      benefit to the patient, are both administered by our
      own medical profession. Do not go anywhere else.

Q. What should I look for in a good *sunscreen?*
A. So many queries are on this topic at the present time
      I am reproducing a list summarising the qualities
      which an ideal sunscreen should possess:

      a It must filter out the rays causing sunburn, which
         are those in the region from 290 to 330 nm.
      b It should be stable in the presence of light, air and
         moisture, or if it is decomposed under these condi-
         tions, the decomposition products should have
         comparable absorption to the original in the 290
         to 330 nm. region.

c It should have very slight or no absorption for the long ultraviolet rays beyond 340 nm., which are thought to produce tanning without appreciable erythema.

d The compound and decomposition products which may be produced under conditions of use should be non-toxic and non-irritating.

e It should be nearly neutral so untoward effects are not produced by the presence of acid or base on the skin.

f It should have good solubility in the ointment base or vehicle in which it is to be formulated and should have a low water solubility to prevent rapid removal by prespiration.

g It should be relatively non-volatile so it will not evaporate under conditions of use.

h It should not be rapidly absorbed by the skin.

Q. I do not know if I feel *tired* because I am depressed or depressed because I am tired and I have been reading a book about health foods and think that I could have some sort of dietary deficiency. Do you think the natural vitamin pills would be better for me as they are much more expensive?

A. Anything is expensive, if it is not the right thing for you. If your diet is deficient in some way it is better to find out in what way this can be remedied from your own Doctor as any attempts at random treatment will at most be ineffective and possibly even hazardous. So, first of all, go to your Doctor and find out. As to the latter part of your question; the health food movement is still extremely controversial and, as in many other areas of dispute, the views of various authorities will often seem to be in conflict. Health elixirs and pills come in an endless variety but heavily advertised products are not always the most potent or effective as the selling price of any

product must, of course, include such high promotion
costs. A healthy discrimination would seem to pay
in this as in most everything else for it is possible
to add many essential nutrients to the daily diet by
the inclusion of staple, inexpensive products.

Q. I have *Vitiligo* and my eyelashes and eyebrows have
virtually no colour at all in them. I use a tint on my
hair and can pencil back my eyebrows but my eyelashes are a never ending trouble to me. I tried false
eyelashes but even after two months cannot seem to
get the knack of applying them and they do not look
right and peel off at the edges. My eyelashes seem
to have thinned out since I started with the false
eyelashes too. I have read about dyes but when I
looked at a bottle, the instructions seemed to be so
complicated that I was too nervous to try it out. What
do you advise me to do?

A. This is a constantly recurring question so let us go
through your problem together, step by step, and it
may well be that others who share them will find some
help too. I note that hair and eyebrows are satisfactory.
I would point out that, however, if you *are* going
to tint your eyelashes, you could do your eyebrows
at the same time and with the same preparation which
would save you the bother and cost of a daily application of eyebrow pencil. Although, theoretically, all
things are possible to all people, to some, some things
are much harder than others and I think that two
months of perseverence indicates that, like many
other people, you find the 'knack' of false eyelash
application too elusive to be feasible in terms of a
busy, everyday routine. You might wish to use them
for special occasions and so the following comments
will help you.

It is possible that your eyelashes look 'wrong'
because you have either, chosen entirely the wrong

shape and type to suit your own eye and face shape or else that, having selected a suitable type of lash you have not trimmed them. As eyelashes are made for average requirements they are usually improved by judicious trimming to fit exactly your own lid and eyeshape. There is, also, a right and wrong way of trimming these. As you do not tell me anything about this, I cannot comment further on this aspect. If your lashes peel off at the edges this could be caused by any or all of the following:

a Grease left on your lid from creams or 'oils'; make sure that your lid is dry and grease-free before applying lashes.

b Failure to apply lash glue evenly along whole length of the eyelash strip before applying.

c Eyelash strip too long for your lid and if this is so, adjust by shortening inside edge of strip.

d Application positioning on lid; centre first and then gently press both sides into place.

False eyelashes, properly applied and removed, are not supposed to diminish your own eyelash growth. In practice, since perhaps, we are not always quite as careful as we should be, I have found that many people from time to time will inadvertently pull out a few of their own lashes too. Now to the question of colourants.

I would suggest that you look at the gel-type *tint,* rather than the liquid type dye, as the former is both gentler in its action and easier to control. Also, that for the first trial, you choose the brown shade. Test first of all, on your fore-arm, but not on your face.

So many people seem to be nervous at the thought of doing this that I have asked Peter to sketch each stage of application for you so that you (and, we hope, a co-operative friend) can think this through, step by step, before you attempt to do it. Finally, judge from your initial reaction, with your patch-test, just how long you are going to leave on the gel, i.e. what depth of colour you want. Set your alarm clock or automatic 'pinger' before you start, so that you can relax *and* be sure that your application will be correctly timed.

Q. I have been told that I should wear a sun cream as I have *Vitiligo.* I have tried out so many creams and spent a small fortune as some of them are very dear. I have not found anything that feels comfortable as they are all so greasy and highly perfumed that I end up feeling like a scented sardine and I just dread the summer coming round again this year. I have read somewhere that if your skin is tanned it is protected against the sun and I am wondering whether I could use an artificial suntan preparation to protect my skin as one or two of these seem to be just clear liquids and it would be lovely to be able to wear something that was not so oily.

A. Lots of questions together, so let's take them one by one. The fake tan colour is produced by a chemical called dihydroxyacetone (DHA). A somewhat complex reaction between DHA and the skin produces a brown pigment but this pseudo-tan colour gives no protection against the sun as would a naturally acquired corporate sunscreen in the self-tan preparations but as these are classed as cosmetics the manufacturers are not compelled to give any indication of the amounts of DHA or protective contained in their products and my advice to you would be to avoid the use of this type of product. Similarly, with chemicals such as sunscreens, you have a right to know what you are putting on your face and should not buy any preparation that does not have the active chemical agent listed on its label or container. The commonly used screening agents can be divided into three groups:

a paminobenzoic acid, generally considered to be the most potent sunscreen.
b benzophenone derivatives
paminobenzoic derivatives such as isoamyl and glycerol
c digalloyl trioleate
cinoxate
menthyl anthranilate
homomenthyl salicylate
triethanolamine salicylate

Screens in this last group offer the least protection of all.

Sunscreen products consist of one of the above types of chemical screens plus its base which may be a lotion, cream, oil, grease or water-alcohol mixture. Although you may not like them, oily and greasy bases are more water-resistant and this is a point you should bear in mind if you are going swimming or are likely to indulge in any heavy outdoor activity and perspire heavily as these bases will stay on better in such conditions but even so these, like any other, should be liberally re-applied after such activities and do remember the often overlooked bits like the sides of your neck and the backs of your hands.

Make-up offers some slight protection but I gather that you do not wish to wear make-up and this means meeting your own ideal requirements with an invisible, non-greasy sunscreen lotion.

Most people can use sunscreen preparations year after year in complete safety but as with most other things, a very small proportion of people will find that certain preparations will produce a sensitivity reaction. If any irritation does occur ever with any preparation you should of course stop using it immediately and report to your Doctor.

I think that it is wrong that you should be there

dreading the approach of summer when it should be a happy time for you and your family. It is so easy to solve the problem and instead of wasting more money on preparations that you do not, or should not, wear I think that you should go back to your Doctor and ask for his advice again. You can sort the problem out once and for all and then you can start looking forward to your summers again.

7: WHERE NOW?

A wound heals through a state of change in the surrounding tissue; a process so common that we give it little, or no thought, and yet the same process takes place in all other parts of the human body: and also the mind. We respond to an insult, to a hurtful remark through a process of mental adjustment, regardless of individual reaction; we make a change within our mind.

Most of these things happen so quickly we feel, afterwards, that nothing has happened and that we are back to normal. Yet, because we are living in a state of time, regardless of our efforts or intentions, we are never able to return to a previous state.

People who suffer from skin damage/disfigurement have a continuous self-awareness of their condition forced upon them through the reactions of other people and will make constant changes from the norm in an effort to adjust to this; changes which, without proper understanding can produce qualities in themselves so different from those of other people, that relating can become extremely difficult and sometimes impossible.

A person with a visual problem will never quite know what it is to live without that problem and a person without such a problem will never quite understand these feelings. The first step towards relating must come from the person who is different; they must understand the nature of other people's reactions and accept, without rancour, that it is not wrong that others should react to something that is not of the ordinary pattern of things. If we see a man with green hair, we look, and take stock of the unusual, processing it in our minds to decide whether it is safe or dangerous, funny or frightening, before relating, or, ignoring it.

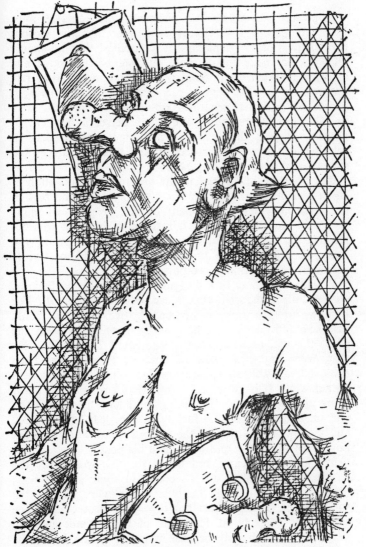

Behind my mask I am a beautiful person.

A person with an obvious disfigurement, similarly, must learn to accept and expect such reactions, in various forms, from other people and it is essential that we should all work to make this a more enlightened, informed and civilised reaction. It is from this point onwards that real progress is possible and, more important, that the self-protective gulf that separates will start to diminish. It is, in fact, by understanding the other person's problem of relating to you, that you will put your own problem of relating into a proper perspective, and so create a relationship of real understanding between you both.

Relationships and creation, the progressive application of effort and mind, are the soul-food of happiness and part of the challenge and achievement of life. If you can make sure that each day has its fair share of both, it will not remove the condition of difference, but it will assure you that you will not be a prisoner of your problem; and to a free person all things are possible.

Perhaps it is only as a disfigured person: badly, facially, congenitally disfigured, that I can write these words. For I know, along with many of you who will read this book, just how hard it is, just how many tears lie between the wish, the will and the accomplishment. I know, like you, that every day is a battle to hold on to what has been achieved, as well as to prepare for what you hope will be achieved. It is because I know, that I set out, so many years ago, to try and alter things and have persevered on and on, most of the time feeling so very lost and helpless; and more than a little like the famous sailor who cried out how large the ocean and how small his boat.

My journey, dreams and hopes for this work over the past forty years have often seemed, in some curious way, comparable to that of the lone sailor who, despite the smallness of his boat, survived the storm protected by the armour of great faith. This kind of faith is not ego and keeps its strength only because it holds, within itself, the essence of truth.

For me, the small boat was the small car. The seas, the many highways and roadways that led me from hospital, meeting to meeting, person to person. But the elements that assailed me and my small car as we drove long into the night to make the next appointment were not only the wind rain and snow but also, the ridicule, contempt, disinterest, mis-understanding and gross cupidity found so often, and all too often, in men and women in all walks of life. Truly, 'none are so blind as those who will not see'.

There were days when it took me all my time to bite back the tears in a confusion of anger and frustration; the cool, indifferent voices, shuffling people and their problems like so many playing cards, would merge with the anxious, worried voices wanting help; . . . the endless 'Yes, it's a good idea. We'll think about it' . . . repeated year after year; the amused receptions, 'We heard you were a mad lady who lived in a car', the plaintive trying-to-be-brave-and-helpful voices of my own beloved son, and twin daughters, 'Oh Mummy, do you *have* to go again?', would all echo and re-echo through my head and conscience as I travelled from place to place. I tried so hard to know and do what was right, but with so many tasks and responsibilities, whatever I was doing would trouble me and it became ever more difficult to decide the priorities of all that needed to be done.

I fretted and worried about the cost it began, increasingly, to demand of others around me and the effort and sacrifice the continuation of these ever-expanding growing activities exacted, also, from my own most wonderful parents who, at a time when they should have been relaxing and enjoying their grandchildren, instead, were washing, ironing, cooking and caring for them. There was the harrassment to us all of the many casual callers to our home and the incessant telephone that would start ringing, often from around 7.00 a.m. and continue until ten or eleven at night, weekends included, and which in our very small house, allowed no peace for anyone and my concern about all these things added to the problem of the sheer physical exhaustion that seemed to overshadow my days.

Often it took years of correspondence, phone calls and visits before I could get a clinic established in an area. Yet, although I was working much, much more than at any full time job, I had no salary, no re-imbursement of any expenses, no assistance towards the hire-purchase or maintenance of a car. There were no funds except those which I could earn and as these were totally non-existent at first and later, so grossly inadequate, related only to the actual clinic hours in hospital, I was forced to pay, out of my own savings, to subsidise the clinics it had already cost so much to obtain; and the more clinics I started, the more it cost me.

My debts started to pile up and travelling became an increasing nightmare. Soon, without money to pay for hotels, the only way I could keep appointments that might be hundreds of miles apart and could not be altered as they had often taken months to arrange, would be to leave home at nine, ten, eleven o'clock and drive through the night, straight to the appointment. Similarly, with many clinics, for, although I usually worked through lunch-breaks and did most of the correspondence at home, it was often seven or eight o'clock at night when I would pack away my things and drive off to the next meeting, wherever that would be.

A breakdown became a terrifying prospect. On two or three occasions, after being involved in accidents and badly knocked about I had to make my car crawl home regardless, as I had no money to pay for help of any kind and, indeed, on one such occasion, frightened everyone, including myself, by arriving home in a pool of blood, to which the scars on my legs still bear testimony.

On my return home, there would be hundred of letters; families desperately in need of guidance; people whose doctors had refused to refer them; doctors who, quite rightly, wanted to be given information about my work before referring their patients; overseas enquiries of many kinds; little children sending me their drawings and dear little letters hoping so hard to get a letter back from me; patients wanting further help, asking if they could call in to see me 'as they were passing'; consultants asking about various, special patients; officials in connection with the training proposals I worked out and submitted in 1969, and all manner of 'administrative' correspondence; often there would be irate letters demanding to know why they had not received an immediate reply but, strangely, rarely thinking to enclose a stamp or even an addressed envelope for same! And always, there would be the letters from my own friends and family saying 'Why don't you write to us any more Doey?' and 'Why haven't you been to see us for such a long time?' No matter how hard I tried, with one pair of hands it became (and still is) increasingly difficult to cope, which of course, added even more to my distress, for I knew, and know, only too well, how anxiously one awaits a reply after having plucked up the courage to write and ask for help.

An appointment for a single patient could often involve me in a protracted correspondence with patient, parents, doctor, hospital, before and after the consultation and this also applies to the many people who had to wait for long periods to obtain an appointment and whose only help whilst waiting was the limited-but-better-than-nothing support of an exchange of letters. Effective and permanent help for some patients entails an initial continuation of the encouragement of the first consultation and in many instances this could only be through correspondence. Stationery and stamp costs began to assume gargantuan proportions and I tried to cope by writing more and more, into the midnight hours, but this, added to the excessive night driving, the worry over ever mounting debts began to take a heavy toll of my eye-sight, appearance and health.

Throughout all the years, the belief, the 'truth' of what

H

I was striving to establish has been like the guiding star to the sailor in his small boat and through all the mockery, deliberate official delays and deceptions, it has never wavered.

For the Society I founded, and myself, and the many patients I have seen over the last two decades, and the patients still waiting for help, the journey is still far from over. The dream of a free, safe, comprehensive, supportive service for disfigurement; of an adequate programme of research and training, and the establishment of a home or centre for use as a base for the proper development of this work, is still a long way from its fulfillment. But I believe with all my heart that, eventually, it will be achieved.

In my own small way I have tried to set down the first few stepping stones across a wide and often treacherous river of ignorance. If now, we each cast a small pebble in this river we will have, soon, a mighty bridge and truly we shall reach the other side; as people, with a disfigurement, but not 'disfigured people'.

Some years ago, a friend gave a book to me. 'I sat up most of the night' she said, 'trying to find the right inscription for you'. I hope that she did. For me, and for all who read this book.

> He said not:
>> Thou shalt not be tempested;
>> Thou shalt not be travailed;
>> Thou shalt not be distressed.
> But He said:
>> Thou shalt not be overcome.
>>> *Julian of Norwich 1317*

GLOSSARY

Some helpful definition explanations

Medical Terminology is unfamiliar to most of us and can be both frightening and confusing. Similarly, various semi-technical, professional references to items or techniques can be perplexing to those who follow different occupations. In the limited space available, I have been guided *only* by the enquiries and queries I have received, over many years and this has produced a somewhat disparate collection of definitions and explanations.

Abscess A cavity which contains pus. In many sites abscess cavities, unless surgically relieved, can enlarge and ultimately rupture onto the surface of the body or into some hollow cavity or organ. Pus can produce a track or infective sinus when discharging from an abscess cavity. An abscess may be acute or chronic.

Acne A term denoting an inflammatory condition of the sebaceous glands.

Acne rosacea Of unknown etiology. A condition in which chronic congestion can lead to enlargement of the minute blood vessels, lumpiness and a red or dusky-copper colour, especially of the nose and in a 'butterfly' shape.

Acne vulgaris A very common disorder amongst teen-agers of either sex. The disease waxes and wanes in intensity and may persist for years and cause considerable psychological disturbance because of its appearance. In-creased secretion of sebum (the oily secretion of sebaceous glands, are features of this condition and the characteristic lesions, blackheads (or comedones), papules, pustules, tiny scars and cysts occur principally on the face, neck, shoulders and upper chest, both back and front. Treatment, which should be under *medical* supervision, can include dietary guidance, Tetracycline orally, Ultra-violet, X-rays and a variety of local treatments to encourage peeling of the skin to enable the sebaceous glands to discharge their contents more readily.

Aetiology   (See Etiology).

Allergen   A substance that stimulates an altered reaction in the body known as an allergy. For example, pollen is the allergen responsible for Hay Fever.

Allergy   Means 'altered reaction'. Sensitivity to various agents which normally produce no adverse reaction but which can, in susceptible individuals, produce a range of clinical disorders. Asthma, hay fever and some types of urticaria and eczema are examples of allergic states. Certain of the effects seen in allergic disorders are due to the liberation of a substance called histamine within the tissues, causing dilation of capillaries, arterioles and venules. In the treatment of allergic disorders such effects may be controlled by the administration of anti-histamine drugs.

Anatomy   Study of normal body structure.

Angioma   An innocent tumour composed of blood vessels.

Antiseptics   Substances which render disease-producing microbes harmless by preventing their growth and multiplication (e.g. surgical spirit, hibitane).

Appendages of the skin   Hair follicles, sebaceous glands and sweat glands together with hair and nails.

Areola   A ring of pigmentation, e.g. as surrounds nipple.

Autopsy   Post mortem examination.

Biopsy   Removal of a small fragment of tissue from living subject, for microscopic examination — frequently under local anaesthetic.

Birthmarks   Present at birth, are of various kinds, the most common being the haemangioma/capillary angioma/naevus fiammens/Port wine stain and pigment spots/moles.

Bullae   Are larger blisters — usually bigger than a pea.

Burrows Are seen only in scabies and are small tunnels made by the female scabies mite, usually in certain characteristic sites.

Capillaries Hair-like, minute vessels connecting arteries and veins and forming a mesh-work all through the tissues of the body.

Carbon Dioxide snow Solidified frozen carbon dioxide, used in the treatment of warts and naevi.

Cellulitis Inflamation of cellular tissue. A severe form of cellulitis is seen in the streptococcal infection called 'erysipelas'. This term is often loosely, and wrongly, used by 'beauty' world.

Cheloid (See Keloid).

Chemexfoliation *(Chemosurgery)* The application of chemicals, such as Phenol, Resorcinal, Trichloracetic acid, to the skin for the purpose of producing an exfoliation to enhance cutaneous improvement (only to be considered when administered by persons holding the proper medical qualification — i.e. Surgeon or Dermatologist — if you value your skin).

Clinical history Facts pertaining to patient's condition.

Comedones Specialised lesions seen in Acne Vulgaris (but commonly called blackheads), small black dots situated at the mouths of hair follicles — often raised on a tiny papule. The black dot is the visible portion of a tiny oval 'plug' in the hair follicle.

Crusts The exudation of serum from the skin surface, which then dries. Crusts stick to the surface and may be straw-coloured or, if mixed with scales, blood or pus, greyish, yellowish or reddish-black. The 'scab' is a crust.

Cutaneous Pertaining to the skin (similarly the prefix 'derm').

Depilatory An agent which will destroy hair (but not the root).

Dermatologist Doctor and Skin Specialist.

Dermatology The study of the skin, its nature, structure, functions, diseases and treatment.

Desquamation Peeling of the superficial layer of the skin.

Diagnosis The recognition and statement of the nature of a particular disease from its symptoms.

Disease Departure from a normal state of health. A condition in which some abnormality of structure or function, or of both structure and function, is present in some part, or parts of the body.

Acquired disease Acquired after birth.

Acute disease Manifested by recent symptoms: of a rapid onset and progress: of a severe or violent nature.

Allergic disease Due to various types of hypersensitivity, e.g. Hay Fever.

Chronic disease Of long duration — slow onset and progress.

Congenital disease Present at birth (to be differentiated from hereditary disease, i.e. inherited).

Contagious disease Spread by direct contact.

Endemic disease One which characteristically occurs in a particular region or locality.

Functional disease Without demonstrable abnormality of structure but associated with abnormality of function.

Iatrogenic disease Meaning 'produced by physicians' arising as a result of treatments administered for other diseases, e.g. reactions from administrations of penicillin.

Local disease Involving only a part of the body (in contradistinction to systemic disease).

Organic disease Associated with structural abnormality.

Silent disease Producing no symptoms or readily detectable signs.

Systemic disease Involving the body (i.e. the system) as a whole.

Disinfectants (Germicides) Substances which destroy pathogenic microbes (e.g. lysol, phenol).

Epilation Removal of hairs with their roots.

Erythema Denotes redness of the skin. It may be localised or generalised. Various causes.

Etiology (also Aetiology) The study of the causes of disease.

Exclamation mark hairs Small stumps of broken hair resembling a printer's exclamation mark, seen at the margin of bald patches on the scalp in alopecia areata.

Exfoliation The separation of dead tissue in thin flaky layers, i.e. shedding of the superficial layers of the skin. Desquamation.

Eye colour Shade of the iris of the eye, such as brown, grey, etc.

Eye shadow colour The deepest natural colour-tone in the eye socket.

Fat-over-lean An ancient and fundamental rule in oil painting (and skin camouflage!). Initial layers should be lean-high pigment, low oil content and the layers above get progressively fatter.

Fissures Cracks which may appear on the skin surface when it is covered with crusts, if it is lichenified or, for any other reason, becomes thickened and inelastic.

Fistula A track with two open ends formed when an abscess bursts and discharges pus in two directions. A fistula may lead from one body cavity to another or lead from skin to mucous membrane.

Haemangioma A tumour of vascular tissue of which there are several forms. Briefly:

Cutaneous Haemanigioma: Port wine Stain/Naevus Flammens/Capillary Angioma (Sturge-Weber Syndrome/Klippel Trenaunay Syndrome)

Strawberry Naevus

Cavernous Haemangioma (Moffuccis Syndrome)

The mixed or combined Haemangioma

The Spider Naevus

Methods of treatment which can be employed:

Conservative

Radiation

CO_2

Injections
Surgery
Steroids
Skin Camouflage and cosmetic masking creams

Haematoma Collection of blood forming a definite swelling. May occur as the result of any injury or operation.

Herpes Simplex 'Cold sores' — a virus infection which causes redness and vesicle formation. It develops most commonly around the mouth. Infectious and once infected the virus persists in the body for the rest of the patient's life. Symptoms vary with age of infection.

Hormones Secretions of ductless glands, and synthetic preparations identical with, or closely resembling, these secretions (e.g. insulin, cortisone, oestrogens) and which, on absorption into the blood, influence the action of tissues and organs other than those in which they are produced.

Ichthyosis Derives from Greek word meaning 'shark skin'. A congenital hereditary abnormality of the skin in which the surface is very rough and presents a dry, cracked appearance resembling fish scales. The skin is permanently hard and deficient in oil and although a warm, sunny climate eases this, in the absence of specific internal treatment, constant external treatment is most important.

Infection Infection is said to be present when disease-producing germs have established themselves and are able to survive and reproduce themselves in the tissues of some part or parts of the body. Infection results in tissue damage and, in the vast majority of cases, shows in the clinical signs and symptoms of infective disease. (The presence of bacteria living on the external and certain internal (e.g. bowel) surfaces of the body does not constitute infection).

Inflammation The local reaction to any form of damage to its cells from infection or other types of injury (e.g.

external physical and chemical agents). There are different types of inflammation but all are essentially defensive in nature.

Keloid (Also Cheloid) An overgrowth of fibrous tissue may result in the production of tumour-like masses in scars. Gets its name from its claw-like off-shoots, which pucker up the surrounding skin. Sometimes these growths disappear spontaneously after a period of activity.

Lesion Word means injury — conveniently employed to refer to any form of structural damage, caused to body tissues by disease.

Leucoderma A condition of the skin in which areas of it become white as a result of various skin diseases or reactions to substances such as the hydroquinone anti-oxidants of rubber goods.

Lichenification The appearance resulting from thickening of the epidermis. The surface of the skin is reddened and covered with fine scales. It feels leathery and inelastic and shows exaggeration of the normal skin folds (like the 'graining' of Morocco leather).

Lip gloss Lubricant shine for use over other lip colours (though now sold coloured as well).

Macules Spots on the skin which can be seen but not felt. They have length and breadth and are flat. The simplest example is a freckle. Macules are usually red, pale or pigmented.

Materia medica Study of drugs used in medicine.

Medium All combinations of ingredients suitable for adding to or combining with paint to affect the consistency and setting times.

Metastasis (Plural: metastases) — secondary lesion of a disease, occurring in a site at a distance from the first centre of disease. Mostly used in relation to malignant disorders, but also with reference to various infective disorders.

Mousseline de soie A fine silk net material used for

simulated face-lift effects. Organza de soie can be used also as a base cover for eyebrows.

Mycosis A disease caused by fungi.

Naevus The term applied to birthmarks consisting of a circumscribed mass of dilated blood vessels. These may take the form of the large port wine stain or occur as swellings of a more restricted nature. *Naevus flammens:* port wine stain. *Naevus pilosus:* A hairy naevus. *Spider naevus:* A small red area surrounded by dilated capillaries. *Strawberry naevus:* Raised tumour-like structure, often regress spontaneously.

Neoplasm Neoplasms — 'new formations' — consist of masses of abnormal cells, which grow at the expense of surrounding normal body tissues and carry out no useful functions in the body. They may be benign (innocent) — e.g. Lipoma — or malignant — e.g. Rodent Ulcer.

Nodules Like papules, but involve the full thickness of skin so that they can be felt not only on the surface but also in the depths of the skin and, even, subcutaneous tissue.

Nose putty Wax putty, theatrical usage for building up facial features. Mortician's wax has a softer consistency.

Paint A combination of pigment and binder to hold or cement the pigment in place.

Papules They can be both seen and felt, i.e. length, breadth and raised. The surface may be rounded, flat-topped or pointed sometimes with an indented or umbilicated depression in the centre. (The common pimple is a papule).

Pharm- Prefix — means 'pertaining to drugs'.

Pharmacology Study of drugs.

Physiology Study of normal body functions.

Pigmentation May be localised, mottled or diffuse, presents as 'discolouration' of various tones of brown, black, yellow.

Prognosis The foretelling of the probable course, duration and outcome of a disease.

Prosthetic Artificial aid for aiding to, changing or replacing natural features and body parts of the anatomy. Constructed of latex, various plastics and many other materials. *Prosthesis* (plural prostheses).

Psoriasis A non-infectious, common disease of unknown origin and chronic course in which reddish, marginated patches with profuse silvery scaling occur in any part of the skin but most commonly over the knees and elbows and in the scalp. The disease is divided into several varieties according to the size, shape and distribution of these patches.

Psychiatry Study and treatment of diseases of the mind.

Psychology Study of the mind.

Purulent Consisting of pus.

Pus A yellowish fluid composed of fluid from the blood, dead and living bacteria, white blood cells and dead tissue cells. It lies initially within a cavity in the tissue which is formed as a result of tissue destruction.

Pustules Skin lesions containing pus. They may start as papules, vesicles or bullae and become pustular or be pustules from their onset. If around a hair, they are called follicular pustules. The Smallpox rash is at first macular, then goes through papular, vesicular and pustular stages.

Pyogenic Producing pus — infections characterised by purulent inflammatory exudates (e.g. Scarlet Fever) are frequently termed 'pyogenic infections'.

Rash ('Eruption'). A superficial eruption on the skin (in lay terms — spots) which may be of, and progress through, various lesions (macule, vesicle, etc.) and usually characterise some specific disease. A rash may be described as petechial, when it is of small purplish spots due to blood effused below the epidermis, called petechiae, or as purpuric when haemorrhages beneath the skin produce large purple spots or patches.

Resolution Return to normal after a disease process.

Rodent ulcer (Basal-cell carcinoma). A carcinoma arising in cells of the epidermis. The face is by far the commonest site for its occurence. Rarely appears before middle age.

Sarcoidosis A relatively rare, chronic disease of unknown origin, in some ways similar to tuberculosis. It involves the skin, lymph nodes, eyes, salivary glands, lungs and bones of feet and hands. In the skin, sarcoidosis may produce a nodular condition called Boecks Sarcoid or more rarely a condition affecting the cheeks and nose called Lupus Pernio.

Scales Dry, silvery-grey flakes of epidermal horn cells which are often seen on the surface of skin lesions where the normal production of cells is altered, e.g. psoriasis or eczema.

Scars The end result of many skin disorders. They may be pin-pointed (e.g. in Acne), irregular, strophic or hyper-trophic (keloid).

Scleroderma A disease marked by progressive hardening of the skin in patches (scleroma) or diffusely with rigidity of the underlying tissues. Often chronic.

Scumbling A scumble is a film of colour laid over another paint surface so that it modifies the original colour but does not completely mask it. (In pure art practice, this is usually a light colour over a darker.) The effect of this is to give a soft, natural 'optical' effect.

Sebaceous glands Minute glands in the skin, situated alongside and opening into the hair follicle a short distance below the point at which the hair emerges on the skin surface. These glands secrete an oily material called sebum These glands are especially large on the nose where their openings are clearly visible.

Sebhorroea A term used to describe an accumulation of excessive secretion of sebum. Commonly occurs on the head and can cause partial hair loss. A form of this disease occurs on the scalp of infants.

Sebum Fatty secretion of the sebaceous glands.

Serum Clear, yellowish fluid which separates from the blood, lymph and other fluids of the body when clotting takes place. The relation of these is shown:

$$\text{Blood} = \left\{ \begin{array}{l} \text{Plasma} - \begin{array}{l} \text{Serum} \\ \text{Fibrin} \end{array} \\ \text{Corpuscles} \end{array} \right\} = \text{Clot}$$

Signs Abnormalities noted by the observer. (Thus the phrase 'signs and symptoms').

Skin camouflage The cosmetic component of disfigurement therapy. The application of preparations to the skin to obliterate temporarily, mute or counterbalance skin damage. Medical approval and consent are a prerequisite for the safe and proper application of skin camouflage techniques.

Skin colour The general colour tone of the face without make-up which will relate to the natural hair colouring. A loose guide only, e.g. medium in a blonde would have a predominance of pink while medium in a brunette would veer to the yellow/olive.

Skin condition Dry, oily, combination, normal, juvenile, etc.

Steroids Group name for compounds which include certain hormones produced in the cortex of the suprarenal glands and called corticosteroids (e.g. cortisone, hydrocortisone) and certain synthetic drugs (e.g. prednisolone) the sex hormones.

Superfatted Having in it more fat than will combine with the alkali present.

Suppuration Formation of pus.

Sycosis Staphylococcal inflammation of the hair follicles, especially those of the beard — sycosis barbae, barber's itch. Characterised by pustules which form into scabs.

Symptoms Abnormalities which are noted by the patient and may indicate the nature and location of a disease, e.g. giddiness, pain.

Syndrome A combination of a number of symptoms which occur together.

Telangiectasis A group of dilated capillaries, web-like or radiating in form. Often seen on the face.

Tinea A skin disease caused by parasitic fungi and named after the area of the body affected, e.g. Tinea capitis: the head. Tinea cruris: the groin.

Tranquillisers Substances which diminish anxiety and excitability by a sedative action on the nervous system (e.g. chlorpromazine).

Tumour In its widest sense, any form of swelling except passing swellings caused by inflammation. The causes of the majority of tumours are still largely undiscovered and they are now classed according to the tissues of which they are built, i.e. simple tumours of normal tissue (Adenoma); hollow tumours or cysts, generally of simple nature; malignant tumours (Cancer and Sarcoma).

Ulcer Is the result of the inflammatory destruction of the full, thickness of the skin or mucous membranes on open sore. It shows a reddish, glistening base, which may be covered with pus or slough. The margin may be oedematous.

Vesicle Is a small watery blister containing clear fluid, i.e. serum. It may start as a papule and progress to a vesicle. Chicken Pox is characterised by a vesicular rash.

Vitiligo A skin disease in which progressive depigmentation produces smooth, white areas on the skin of the face and body. There is sometimes a marked loss of pigment from the hair.

Weals Are caused by oedema of the full thickness of the skin and are raised red lumps varying in size, with an ill-defined margin often with a pale centre. The characteristic lesions of urticaria (nettle rash), hives or heat lumps.

Wound Gap in an external or internal body surface caused by injury.